A NEW YOU IN 21 DAYS

Bronwen Meredith

A NEW YOU IN 21 DAYS

Elm Tree Books . London

First published in Great Britain 1983
by Elm Tree Books/Hamish Hamilton Ltd
Garden House 57-59 Long Acre London WC2E 9JZ

Book design by Paul Bowden
Illustrations by Edward Cairns
Weekly exercise plans by Andy Ingham

British Library Cataloguing in Publication Data

Meredith, Bronwen
    A new you in 21 days.
    1. Beauty, personal   2. Women—Health and
    hygiene
    I. Title
    646.7'088042   RA778

    ISBN 0-241-10948-5
    ISBN 0-241-10949-3 Pbk

Filmset by Pioneer
Printed and bound in Great Britain by
Redwood Burn Ltd, Trowbridge, Wiltshire

CONTENTS

A NEW YOU...

HOW REALISTIC?

Every woman can be good looking . . . it is only a matter of gaining knowledge, sparing time and putting in effort: most of all — will-power.

21 days can bring about a remarkable change . . . in weight, shape, fitness, general attitude and beauty, but only if you are prepared to follow a constructive plan.

You can look great at any age . . . once you learn the disciplines, the routines, the building bricks for health, the tricks for the most successful image.

There are five ways to a NEW YOU . . .
- give up laziness — take exercise, start sport
- give up overeating — watch your diet, judge foods
- give up bad habits — cut out smoking and drinking
- give up apathy — make an effort to be beautiful
- give up negativeness — you can do anything, be anyone

Give 21 days to positive health and beauty . . . you'll be amazed at the improvement, at the results, at the difference in your feelings, your attitude, your looks, not to mention the difference in other people's reactions to you. It's all planned out right here. A page a day and you're well on your way. Turn over . . . and CHECK IN

CHECK IN

How do you shape up? Are you really interested in looking better, in changing bad habits? Here is a quick questionnaire to check on your attitude towards health and beauty — and to establish whether you are doing anything positive towards looking better and feeling fitter.

DIET

Do you watch your food intake?

Have you any idea how many calories you consume a day?

Are you conscious of what constitutes healthy eating?

Have you ever really stuck to a diet before?

Have you the will-power to give up all alcohol?

Do you ever think of eating fruit in place of dessert, cake or sweets?

EXERCISE

Do you walk a fair amount each day?

Do you participate in any outdoor activity — cycling, jogging, a sport?

Have you previously followed a regular exercise regime?

Do you know which movements are best for specific body areas?

Are you full of energy with enough stamina for anything?

Do you consider yourself at a peak of fitness?

SKIN CARE

Do you know your skin type and how to care for it?

Do you have a daily skincare programme you follow religiously?

Do you ever do anything specific for special problems?

Do you really know what each skincare product does?

Have you ever given yourself a facial at home?

Do you pay as much attention to your body skin as that on your face?

BODY CHECK

Have you ever had a complete physical checkup?

Do you know your blood pressure, your blood group?

Do you regularly check up for cancer through breast examination and cervical smear test?

Have you visited the dentist within the last year? The optician? The chiropodist?

Do you know ways of relaxation or ways to help stress?

BEAUTY POINTER

Are you absolutely happy with the way you look?

Do you make the most of your face?

Are you up to date with the latest cosmetics and the ways of applying them?

Do you use brushes when you make-up?

Have you changed your hairstyle over the last 2 years, had a new cut, altered colour?

Do you regularly have your hair cut?

Do you do anything yourself to condition your hair?

Do you constantly check in magazines for new ideas, new looks, new images?

Do you manicure your nails every week?

Do you think of perfume as a daily essential?

OPTIONAL

Have you had a professional facial treatment within the last year?

Does it ever occur to you to have a regular massage?

Have you considered joining a club or gym for an exercise programme?

Do you have a salon pedicure each month?

Do you know anything about aromatic treatments?

Have you allowed yourself a complete day of rest recently?

Have you treated yourself to something really marvellous within the last 6 months — something to wear, something for beauty?

PERSONAL DATA

Weight: _____	General fitness:	Good ___ Much Improved ___ The Same ___
Measurements:	Figure:	Good ___ Much Improved ___ The Same ___
Bust _____	Diet habits:	Good ___ Much Improved ___ The Same ___
Waist _____	Skin condition:	Good ___ Much Improved ___ The Same ___
Hips _____	Make-up:	Good ___ Much Improved ___ The Same ___
Thighs _____	Hair condition:	Good ___ Much Improved ___ The Same ___
Knees _____	Hairstyle:	Good ___ Much Improved ___ The Same ___
Calves _____	Hands and nails:	Good ___ Much Improved ___ The Same ___
Upper arms _____	Emotional state:	Good ___ Much Improved ___ The Same ___

If you've answered 'NO' to most of these questions, then it's about time you started paying more attention to yourself. It is not vain to pursue a better looking you — it's an essential way to build up confidence. If you slowly learn the basics of health and beauty, and apply them day by day, you'll see startling results in a few weeks. Start now, start here . . .

DAY TO DAY PLAN

How it works:

An outline is given on what to do each day. It is so planned that all aspects of this health and beauty regimen are done in logical sequence. You are first given the basics and then build on that, expanding to greater demands on your body, more finesse with your beauty. It's a gradual construction, so follow each day as suggested. Do no more — and please do no less. If you don't pay heed one day, you may not be able to cope with the next. There are 6 points to check on.

DIET

This is specifically set for each day and should be followed as stated. Sometimes extras are included such as drinks and juices to liven up the day. There are also cooking tips, guides on vitamins and minerals, plus notes on the special value of certain foods and herbs. The diet is also printed as a chart: stick it right away on the door of the refrigerator.

EXERCISE

There are 3 phases — a different regime for each of the weeks. The first plan provides relatively easy movements to break you gradually into the habit of daily exercise. The following week the exercises require increased stamina and ability, while the final week presents a still more vigorous series. This last programme is laid out on a wall chart — you can pin it up and continue doing exercises for ever. There are also daily tips and extra movements for specific areas.

SKIN CARE

A day to day build-up so that at the end of 21 days you know all that is necessary for great skin. First you check on type, then learn the routine of basic care. Then on to special treatments, problems and notes on both commercial preparations and home-made ones. Plus a comprehensive wall chart on 'Skincare' designed to hang in your bathroom. It shows the rules of how to clean your face properly, plus a step-by-step guide to the perfect make-up. It will be right in front of your eyes all the time, so there'll be no excuse for not looking marvellous.

BODY CHECK

In turn, all parts of the body are discussed from both the health and beauty angle — fitness, surface condition, specific problems and possible ways for improvement. There are guidelines on legs, hands, feet, breasts, neck, ears, eyes, teeth. Plus a look at emotions — how to relax, how to help stress.

BEAUTY POINTER

The aesthetic side of the New You . . . how to make the most of your visual appeal. There are instructions on how to get the most successful make-up, the best face, with information on products and technique. Then there's hair — views on style, condition and care. And quite a lot of words and tips on perfume.

OPTIONAL

In this section there are suggestions on the more indulgent side of health and beauty — nothing absolutely necessary, but all the things you've probably wanted to do but considered too extravagant. There are suggestions about treatments in salons, by beauty specialists; notes on the value of clubs, of various therapies.

DIET

Breakfast:
½ grapefruit
1 boiled egg
1 slice whole-grain toast
coffee or tea

Lunch:
2 slices cold chicken or turkey (no skin)
1 tomato
6 slices cucumber
as much watercress as you like, seasoned with
  lemon juice and pepper
1 slice whole-grain toast
coffee or tea

Dinner:
125g (4 oz) grilled fish — no butter, seasoned
  with tarragon and lemon
large green salad — lettuce, green peppers,
  cucumber, celery — dressing of cider
  vinegar and one teaspoon olive oil, ground
  pepper and a pinch of salt
coffee or tea

Rules to establish now and continue throughout 21-day regime: no sugar, minimum salt, no butter, use margarine and oil only when indicated. Milk allowance per day is 2 table-spoons skimmed milk or 1 tablespoon full milk. No alcohol or soft drinks but try to drink 575 ml (1 pint) or more of water a day, before or between meals rather than with them. Start every day with the juice of one lemon in warm water (not boiling). Tea and coffee can be drunk anytime, but begin to explore herbal teas (see page 59) they are very beneficial for health and also help to bring some variety to beverages.

BEAUTY POINTER

Is your make-up in order? We are all guilty of hanging on to old tubes and bottles, eye and lipstick colours that are out of date. Throw out all the dead wood and put your make-up into

OPTIONAL

How strong willed are you about exercise? Not very? You are not alone; most women find it very difficult to get down to exercising at home. Those streamlined personalities who say they spend so much time working out and shaping up each day are usually doing it in a gym. The most basic luxury of all is to treat yourself to exercise classes — and not one that meets once a week. Go every day and you'll be forced to put your body through the paces. Clubs and gyms usually have arrangements for weekly and monthly membership. If you can afford it, it is definitely worth every penny. It's a bonus — but still try to follow the exercise plan at home as well.

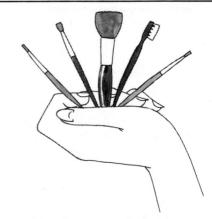

better shape. Keeping it all tidy and handy is essential. A cutlery tray makes a good make-up kit, so does a basket, a sewing box. You don't need nearly as much make-up as you think, particularly now that the desired look is a natural neutral face rather than one of extreme colour. What you do need is a set of brushes, the vital tools of a professional make-up. You can buy sable paintbrushes from any art shop, or you can get sets of cosmetic brushes. These are the ones you'll need — and keep them scrupulously clean, otherwise your skill at using them will be wasted.

EXERCISE

Make up your mind that you are going to do two things; 1. get outdoors and put your whole body into action; 2. discipline yourself to a concentrated period of 20 minutes a day working at specific exercises. For overall conditioning — walk. Nothing's easier. Walk as briskly as you can and on this first day aim to walk 2.5 kilometres (1½ miles) in 30 minutes. For your body work-out, follow the 'First Week Exercise Plan' on page 64. You need space, you need air (open the window). An exercise leotard helps to put you in the right mood, but it's not absolutely necessary. You can exercise in a swimsuit, in your underwear, in the nude. You can't, however, exercise in any constricting clothes. Your body needs freedom to move.

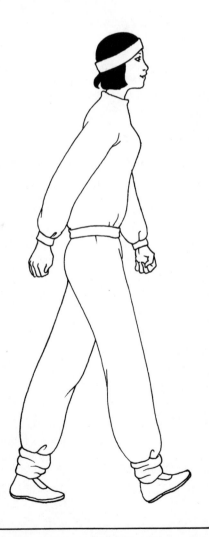

SKIN CARE

Clear your skin of all debris. Even if you are following a regular skincare process, chances are you still have a collection of dry, dead cells on the surface. Do it the way it's done in leading health spas. All you need is a face cloth and some ordinary fine kitchen salt. Soak the cloth in warm water, sprinkle salt all over it and gently rub your entire face. Don't rub hard, gentle circular movements are just as effective. Then rinse away the salt in clear, cool water. Rinse until there's no trace of salt. Feel your skin. Isn't it smooth? It may look a little red, but that soon disappears. Your skin is now able to breathe and looks more alive. Simply smoothe in a moisturizer and don't put on any make-up for a couple of hours. Your entire body can be treated to a salt rub down — rinse away under a cool invigorating shower. It makes you feel good, healthy and pristine clean.

BODY CHECK

Superfluous hair is unsightly no matter where it is. Many women only concern themselves with underarms and legs below the knee. You need a more thorough check than that. Do it today. For details of methods of hair removal, see page 80. The body zones to check on are: face — tweeze the odd, stray hair and tidy up the eyebrows; bleach, wax or use a depilatory for upper lip, electrolysis however is the only permanent method. For underarms, shaving is standard because it is fast and simple, waxing can hurt a lot, but depilatories are fine. Bleaching or waxing is best for arms, depilatories next, never shave. On the breasts you can tweeze out the odd hair, but never from the nipple (snip those) and all other methods are out. Finally the legs — waxing is superior, particularly at the bikini line, shaving is quick but hairs can grow back fast and spiky, depilatories work well, and if you don't have too many hairs, just bleach them.

DIET

Breakfast:
½ grapefruit
toasted cheese on 1 slice whole-grain toast
coffee or tea

Lunch:
fruit salad — 1 orange, 1 apple, 1 slice
   pineapple or melon, 1 banana, a few grapes
   plus the juice of a lemon
2 tablespoons cottage cheese
coffee or tea

Dinner:
125g (4 oz) lean steak
1 cup brussels sprouts or broccoli
lettuce and tomato salad
1 slice whole-grain toast
1 apple or orange
coffee or tea

It has to be mentioned, though it should go without saying to anyone interested in a new fit healthy body, that all foods in the diet must be fresh. Nothing frozen, nothing tinned, nothing packaged. You don't have to buy it everyday because most items will keep perfectly well in the refrigerator. And your bread must be whole-grain, which is widely available or you can make your own (see recipe page 60). Of course, no butter on the bread.

SKIN CARE

Have you got basic care right? No matter what type of skin you have, it needs to be thoroughly cleansed and treated every day. When you do it doesn't matter. Whether you take your make-up off at night or in the morning is irrelevant. You can, of course, go through your skin routine more than once a day — that depends on your personal preferences and lifestyle. However, one precise procedure is adequate and more than 3 times a day is silly because too much attention can cause problems. You need 3 products: a cleanser, a toner, a moisturizer, plus cotton wool — check if you have them. For cleansing, soap and water still takes a lot of beating, and although most mild soaps are fine, the best are the non-alkaline soaps now called 'facial soaps' or 'soap bars'. They are expensive, but because you only use them on your face, they last for ages. If you use soap, you will need a cleanser or a simple oil (almond or baby oil work perfectly) to take off eye make-up. If you don't want to buy a special toner, ordinary witch hazel is excellent and is available at any chemist. A moisturizer is essential and a good one is well worth the money. Consult the 'Skincare Chart' for details on daily care, pin it up in your bathroom — it will be a constant reminder of what you should be doing daily for a great looking skin.

BODY CHECK

Moments of complete relaxation are as important as those of activity. Learning to relax and to let go is a good way to combat stress and tension. Today try the classic Yoga slant: lie in a backward slope with head on the ground and feet raised 30 cm (12 inches) above the floor. Use a firm board — a plank covered with a towel is ideal, but you can also adjust an ironing board to the correct angle. At this angle the spine straightens out and muscles are relaxed, losing all tension. Close your eyes, arms at sides and lie there for 15 minutes. You can use this slant to revive you after a day's work or before going out — it's a quick trick for recovery.

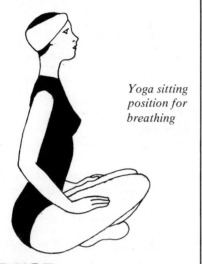

Yoga sitting position for breathing

OPTIONAL

Seek out a health food shop and really get to know the kind of products they sell. You'll find all types of food, an array of vitamin and mineral supplements, many preparations for skin and hair and usually a selection of books. Treat yourself to a few items — a book on the value of Vitamin E, a jar of rare honey to save for later (it's not allowed during the 21-day diet), some multiple vitamin B capsules to take now and a natural conditioning cream to pamper your skin.

EXERCISE

How was the walk yesterday? Do the same today, same speed, same distance. And the exercises? Maybe you feel a little stiff this morning, but run through the whole sequence again and you'll find muscles will ease. Most important — are you breathing properly? You probably haven't even thought about it, because it is such a natural, automatic function. Breathing in deeply is the first rule, but it's during exhalation that most errors occur. Very few of us actually empty our lungs of all the stale air. Test yourself: stand with hands gently on your ribcage. Take a deep breath through your nose, feeling the expansion of the ribcage, the swelling of the abdomen. Now exhale slowly through the nose, using your stomach muscles to push all the air up and out. Really force out the last bit of it — you'll also feel the ribcage drawing together. Good breathing mobilizes lungs and abdomen. It is also a source of energy. Try this Yoga breathing exercise and make it a daily habit: sit down cross-legged, rest hands on thighs, spine straight, head high; breathe in through the nose, hold it to the count of five, then slowly exhale, releasing air by jerking the abdomen — don't let go of all the air at once, jerk, pause, jerk again until lungs are empty. Repeat 5 times.

BEAUTY POINTER

Take a realistic look at your face. Are you happy with your image? Is it time for a change? Keeping your looks up to date with fashion involves being aware of even the subtlest changes. Maybe you've allowed yourself to stay with the same old look for years. A complete make-over is not only great for morale, but can give you a surprising view of the possibilities of a new you. First move is to go out and buy the most stylish magazines. Take your time and leisurely study the looks for now — appraise the ideas in both the editorial and the advertisements within the framework of your face, your hair, your life. And be sensible about your limitations. Cut out the looks that appeal to you and make a 'Personal Beauty' file. These clippings will be invaluable when you go to the hairdresser, want to find a different make-up or experiment with colours. Also if you don't snip them out, you'll forget about them and then throw the magazine away. Keeping such a file is good discipline and encourages you to keep an interest in your looks — and keep up with the new.

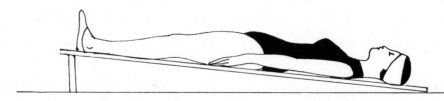

BODY CHECK

A look at legs — or would you rather not? The length and shape of the leg is hereditary and cannot be altered, but fat and loss of muscle control can. Unfortunately thighs tend to accumulate fat that is hard to get rid of. Legs by nature are dry, so today smooth in a skin lotion and remember to do it regularly in the future. Legs often have lazy circulation — one reason for fat accumulation — improve it by vigorously rubbing thighs for 5 minutes with a loofah or a friction glove. Continue to do it daily while bathing. Legs need toning and any force of water is good; alternate hot and cold blasts from the hand shower help firm flesh. And try this exercise to firm thighs: leaning against a wall, feet about a foot away from it, get into a sitting position, back straight, knees at right angles — hold to the count of 5 at first and over the days increase the count to hold as long as possible.

DIET

Breakfast:
2 slices pineapple
1 slice whole-grain toast scraped with
   margarine
coffee or tea

Lunch:
150g (6 oz) fillet of fish, grilled (eat any skin)
1 cereal-bowl of green salad — such as lettuce,
   cress, peppers, cucumber plus onion,
   seasoned with lemon or cider vinegar, a
   teaspoon of vegetable oil, half a pinch of salt
   and much pepper
coffee or tea

Dinner:
150g (6 oz) roast chicken, no skin
cucumber and tomato salad, lemon and
   pepper
½ grapefruit
coffee or tea

The issue of dieting can be very confusing because there seem to be, indeed are, many conflicting regimens. Which one is right, which is the best? Even the experts disagree. Some say it's only the calories that count. Others say quantity doesn't matter but the type of food does, particularly when certain foods are eaten together. This 21-day diet is based on 3 factors: restricting the number of calories, drastically cutting down fats, and balancing the combination of certain types of food.

OPTIONAL

It is well worth seeking out a sauna — clubs, pools, gyms and some beauty salons have them. Having a sauna not only aids the loss of pounds and inches, but encourages the elimination of toxic matter. A sauna is a wood slatted cubicle of very high dry heat. At first it is stifling and even the slats are too hot to sit on without a towel. It is usual to stay in for 10 minutes; afterwards a cold plunge or cool shower is recommended. It is the change from heat to cold that is a significant factor as it stimulates circulation and heart activity. Don't take a sauna until an hour after eating — and if you have any blood pressure problems don't take one at all.

BEAUTY POINTER

Is your hair right? If hair's wrong, it immediately detracts from any other good points. Hair is the great confidence-giver and goes a long way to establishing your personal style. Hair needs to be cut and shaped by a professional, so make an appointment to go to the hairdresser as soon as possible. But go armed with your own ideas — take those clippings, have some definite views in mind. Hairdressers can be terrible bullies — haven't you ever come out of a salon furious at what's been done? So be firm, but you must have suggestions. Move your hair around to see what direction works best for your face. Fiddle with it, pull it back, to one side, over the forehead, up, down and so on. Think about shape, texture, pattern and colour. What needs to change? What can be changed? (see page 94 for hair types and change procedures). Remember it's best to have a style you can easily take care of yourself.

EXERCISE

Continue with the daily walk and daily exercise routine. Rethink posture. Do you realise that good posture gives a better figure instantly? In fact its influence goes further. Many figure problems have their origin in faulty posture. The way you carry and move your body effects its shape. Check how you stand: think tall, imagine a thread pulling you up tautly, stretch the spine and the back of your neck, lower the shoulders easily, pull in stomach, tuck buttocks under; beware of pulling the shoulders too far back and arching the spine. Check how you walk: movement should come from the thighs not hips; don't stick buttocks out or lean forward, keep back straight as you go up and down hill, up and down steps, relax arms allowing them to swing naturally — and walk with a spring, it looks young and vital. Do this exercise to be aware of body alignment: kneel sitting on heels, arms at sides, back straight but relaxed, head inclined a little forward; rise slowly to kneeling position, pulling arms up over the head, stretching spine and neck; hold to the count of 5. Return to heel position, using thigh muscles for lowering. Repeat ten times.

SKIN CARE

This is facial-skin inspection day. Not just the usual look, but a real thorough going over to find out what your skin is about, what's good, what's bad. It is essential to do this in direct daylight and better still to do it with a magnifying mirror even though blemishes appear terrifyingly larger than life. Skin types are confusing. In magazine articles and advertisements they are over-simplified as 'dry' or 'oily'. Actually most skins are a combination of both. Then there's colour to consider which greatly effects texture and performance, and of vital significance is condition — how sensitive, how blemished? So look at your skin bearing all these points in mind. First, cleanse it completely, rinse with cool water, then examine. You can easily see blemishes on your clean skin. You'll also be able to detect coarse and enlarged pores which indicate oily areas, while tight, flaky surfaces inclined to little lines are the result of dry skin. Do you have too many lines for your age and where? Any sign of spider veins? More freckles, new moles? (For details on skin types and problems see page 77.) The first time you properly study your facial skin will most likely be a revelation — and not too pleasant a one at that. But it will put you in contact with what's going on. You'll be more aware of any improvement, more concerned if something goes wrong.

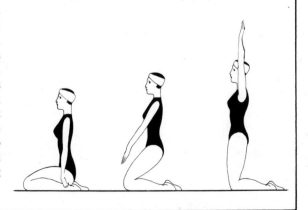

SKIN CARE

Bathing — the first act of beauty — is a daily essential. But do you make the most of it? A morning shower is stimulating and gets you going; make the final rinse as cold as you can bear it; it will tone and help firm the skin. A bath is relaxing and it can soothe and nourish the skin. Check now to see if you have the bath essentials: a mild soap . . . a loofah or friction strap for rubbing off skin, boosting circulation . . . flannel or bath mit (regularly washed, please) . . . 2 body brushes, a long-handled one for your back, a small one for hands and feet . . . pumice stone or synthetic friction block to soften and rub away hard skin. If your skin is dry, an oil becomes an essential, but you can make up your own by adding 1 tablespoon of any liquid detergent shampoo to 1 cup of any kitchen oil and to this add ½ teaspoon of any aromatic oil (from healthfood shop or specialist chemist); pour the mixture into a bottle and shake well before using. You'll need 2 tablespoons per bath. An all-over body lotion helps all skins, but is an absolute must for dry ones.

OPTIONAL

Go to a salon for a facial treatment. It is both a skin and a psychological boost. A skin specialist will analyse your skin, professionally determine its type and texture and suggest suitable skincare products and procedures. Your skin will be cleared of surface debris, blackheads and whiteheads taken out, impurities brought to the surface. It is really an extension of your own basic care routine. It is usual for your face to be gently massaged. Masks range from simple tightening ones to oil and aromatic treatments; sometimes your face is steamed, sometimes drastically cooled, sometimes stimulated with electrical currents — it all depends on the salon. Facials last about an hour and you lie down, relaxed with the therapist working from behind. Faces react in different ways; you may come out looking as though you've been away for a week, or your skin may be stimulated into redness and blotches due to the elimination of toxic matter — this gradually disappears. Results from a facial are temporary, but taken regularly it's a great beauty bonus.

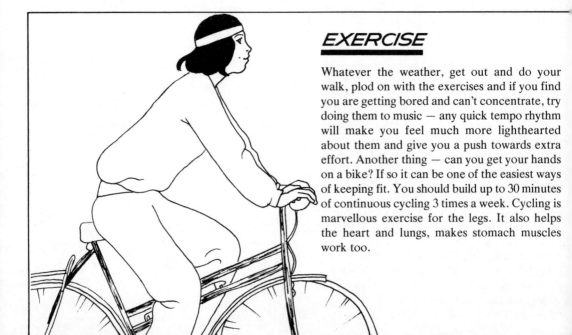

EXERCISE

Whatever the weather, get out and do your walk, plod on with the exercises and if you find you are getting bored and can't concentrate, try doing them to music — any quick tempo rhythm will make you feel much more lighthearted about them and give you a push towards extra effort. Another thing — can you get your hands on a bike? If so it can be one of the easiest ways of keeping fit. You should build up to 30 minutes of continuous cycling 3 times a week. Cycling is marvellous exercise for the legs. It also helps the heart and lungs, makes stomach muscles work too.

DIET

Breakfast:
1 sliced orange
1 boiled egg
1 slice whole-grain toast
coffee or tea

Lunch:
1 omelet using 1 egg, a little milk and a
    smudge of margarine in the pan
1 cup sliced, boiled courgettes
1 slice whole-grain toast
coffee or tea

Dinner:
3 slices boiled or roasted chicken, without skin
1 cup coarsely chopped spinach
1 cup sliced string beans
1 apple
coffee or tea

Water retention can be responsible for some excess pounds and many women retain more water than they need particularly prior to menstruation. There is a lot of water in the body, and proportions are carefully regulated, and one of the chief things that controls the balance is salt. If too much salt is taken, water accumulates with it, tissues swell and you weigh more. We only need about one gramme of salt a day to maintain a healthy water level. Most of us consume 10 or 20 times that much. So watch it. Use little salt. Don't take diuretic pills — they can become a habit and too many are dangerous. Between meals munch on chunks of raw cucumber or celery, and drink lots and lots of water — oddly enough this helps to take away any excess trapped in cells.

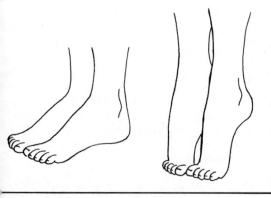

BEAUTY POINTER

If you've been studying your magazine clippings on new faces, you'll be anxious to go out and buy a whole fresh set of make-up products. But hang on, wait. Don't rush before you plan exactly what you need. You'd probably have most items already and there's no need to overstock. Essentials are: foundation, colourless powder, blusher, eyeshadow, eyebrow pencil, mascara and lipstick. (Check page 88 for the different types.) Settle on a basic colour scheme. Foundation should match your skin tone; eyeshadow is best in neutrals such as greys or browns, or low-key colours — it should draw attention to the eyes, not to the colour of the shadow. Blusher and lipstick colours should complement each other. You may also want a cover-up cream, an additional foundation shade for contouring, a choice of eyeshadows, a set of coloured crayons. Make a list and trim it as much as possible. It's skill that counts in make-up not a vast array of products — in fact too many items can cause too much confusion. And you should have your box and brushes organized from Day 1. So get your clippings, list and colour choices sorted out for a shopping spree tomorrow.

BODY CHECK

Have you ever bothered to pay attention to your feet except when they hurt? Four out of five adults finally have foot trouble caused by badly fitting shoes and neglect of basic care. Are all your shoes comfortable? Do you wear low heels for your daily walk? Do you scrub regularly with a pumice stone to prevent build-up of hard skin? Feet need to breathe — do you walk barefoot as often as possible? Examine your feet for corns, bunions and callouses. If you have them, don't try and treat them yourself, but go to a chiropodist. In fact your feet should really go for annual checkups as most foot ailments don't cure themselves, but get worse — and if your feet hurt it shows on your face. Do you know that feet have to be exercised? If they are not, muscles slacken and they have trouble taking the body weight and supporting the bones. Here's a simple exercise to do every day. Stand straight, feet pointing ahead, then raise yourself high on to the ball of the foot, hold to the count of 5, lower. Repeat 10 times.

BODY CHECK

A well turned ankle has always been considered an asset. How fare yours? Some women have naturally fleshy or sturdy ankles and no amount of attention or care can alter them. Usually in this case, though ample, the flesh is firm. If flesh is flabby it can be helped by this exercise: classic foot circles — sit with legs stretched out in front, arch the foot and make wide circles outward. Repeat 10 times. Now make inward circles — 10 times. Do you ever suffer from swollen ankles? These are due to the rules of gravity: blood and body fluids fight against it to return to the heart. Some of the fluid can seep into the tissue around the ankles and puff them up. This can happen when you've been on your feet all day, when shoes or stockings are too tight or when a shift in hormone balance during the premenstrual period or in pregnancy causes fluid retention. Ways to help: rest with feet higher than the rest of the body — the swelling will go down but it may take an hour; rub with ice-cubes; soak feet and ankles in an Epsom salts bath.

OPTIONAL

One of the most pleasurable body and beauty procedures is a massage. It relaxes you, relieves tension through touch. It helps reduce aches and pains. It doesn't, however, break up fatty tissue or reshape the body. But by improving circulation it tones skin and helps toxic elimination. Most important — it makes you conscious of your own body and its potential. You certainly feel slimmer and better — try and see. It's best to have massage after exercise or late in the afternoon when tension is invariably at its peak. Massage is the greatest tranquillizer. There are several ways of giving a massage and masseurs vary enormously in their touch and technique. Stroking and kneading may be light or heavy; circular movements are often included. You will be massaged in the nude; a bland oil or emollient is used. Thirty or forty minutes is the average time.

DIET

Breakfast:
½ grapefruit
toasted cheese on 1 slice whole-grain toast
coffee or tea

Lunch:
1 cup cottage cheese
1 large bowl green salad — add some spinach
  leaves
1 slice whole-grain toast
coffee or tea

Dinner:
125g (4 oz) grilled fish, no skin, seasoned with
  herbs, smeared with a small dab of
  margarine
1 large bowl green salad (same as for lunch)
1 slice whole-grain toast
coffee or tea

Raw vegetable juices are extremely valuable as a concentrated form of vitamins and minerals. You can add a mid-morning drink to your daily diet of the following mixed juice: put 2 cups of carrot juice in the blender and add any available greens, chopped — you can use cabbage, lettuce, parsley, spinach, kale, broccoli — and whisk until thoroughly blended.

EXERCISE

Increase your walk mileage today, aim to walk 3 kilometres (1¾ miles) in 30 minutes. Don't rush your exercises, do them precisely and slowly. Check on everyday movements. Are you walking whenever you can — to the office, to the shops? Are you avoiding the bus, leaving the car in the garage? Are you making yourself run upstairs? Are you doing household tasks briskly instead of dragging your feet around? Do you ever think of taking an extra stroll just for the pleasure of it? Become more aware of every bit of activity.

BEAUTY POINTER

Got your make-up list? Got your magazine clippings? Off you go for a fun day cosmetic shopping. Well, it should be, but many obstacles will be put in your way. Watch out for pushy salesladies and don't be talked into buying anything you don't really want. Watch out for lighting — under artificial light colours change drastically and once home you could get quite a shock at what you selected. Watch out for the sample units, check them all — testers are there for testing, so use them. Watch out for prices, there's no need to buy the most expensive, it's better to spend your money on skincare treatments. Watch out most of all for the perfect foundation; it's the base, the canvas for the rest. Find one that is as close as possible to your skin tone and beware of shades that have too much pink in them. Only wear a moisturizer when foundation-shopping. Try the base on a small area of your face and go into the daylight to check it. And don't let the assistant talk you into putting the foundation on the back of your hand — or worse on hers — to judge the shade. It just doesn't work. To find the right one is a case of trial and error, so persevere.

SKIN CARE

Lines on the face and neck can be helped by gentle stroking. Learn these 4 movements and use them when applying your moisturizer or a conditioning night cream. Try and do them for 5 minutes, and then put in extra time during the day when you are lying in the bath, watching TV. Facial stroking is very light and is done with the tips of the fingers — they should skim across the surface, don't pull or push.

1. Cheeks and mouth — purse lips into an O-shape. With the first, second and third fingers, stroke upwards from the outer corners of the mouth in a V direction up and across the cheeks. Slowly stroke 6 times.
2. Chin and mouth — lips again in an O-shape, with the tips of the first, second and third fingers, stroke upward from the centre of the chin out to the hollow cheeks. Do 6 times.
3. Forehead — mouth normal and closed. With tips of second, third and fourth fingers, start at the centre and work outwards in a circular movement drawing to the centre again at the top. Repeat 6 times.
4. Throat and chin — mouth closed, use first, second and third fingers to trace a course upward from the collar bone to the tip of the chin. Repeat 6 times.

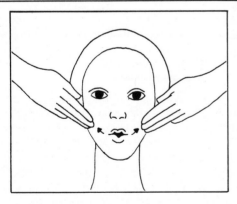

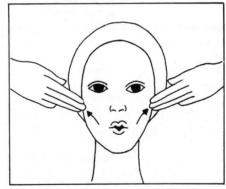

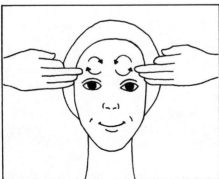

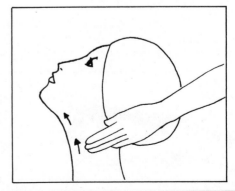

DAY 6

DIET

Breakfast:
1 slice melon
1 slice whole-grain toast
coffee or tea

Lunch:
1 large bowl of fruit salad, any fruit you like,
  sprinkled with the juice of a lemon
½ cup cottage cheese
coffee or tea

Dinner:
2 slices breast of chicken or turkey, no skin
1 sliced tomato, plus 8 slices cucumber
1 slice whole-grain toast
1 apple or orange
coffee or tea

Vitamins are essential in every diet because
they regulate body functions. They are not body
builders, nor do they provide energy. They are
more like directors — they organize metabolism
and occasionally take part themselves. Vitamins
can help you resist disease and it is now believed
that they are our best protection against
environmental stress and pollutants. Most of
the vitamins we need come from the vegetable
and fruit carbohydrate foods. This 21-day diet
is balanced for essential vitamin intake. If you
like you can take a compound of vitamins B-1,
B-2 and B-6 which aids digestion, a compound
of vitamins A, D, E and F for the skin, and
vitamin C (2 grammes a day) to help ward off
colds, to combat stress and build up resistance
to infections.

SKIN CARE

Look at the skin on your hands. It is one of your
most vulnerable areas, and needs daily care as
much as your face. There is one simple rule:
lots of cream. This will hold in the moisture and
prevent chapping, rough skin and cracks. The
more you cream your hands the better. Any
lotion will do, you can even use something as
ordinary as vaseline. Hands will soak it up.
Wipe off any excess with a tissue. You can
make your own handcream:

150g (6 oz) lanolin
 75g (3 oz) honey
 75g (3 oz) almond oil

Melt the lanolin in a double boiler, cool a little,
add the honey and whisk until thoroughly
blended — by hand or in a blender. Finally, stir
in the almond oil, drop by drop, and beat until
smooth. Put in an airtight container.

EXERCISE

On with your faster walk, on with those
exercises. At this point you need to learn how
to put your body in a restful position, but helping
its shape at the same time. Again a Yoga
discipline is the answer. It's called 'The Pose of
a Child' and is a restful asana (posture), a
constructive way of relaxing the body after a
strenuous exercise or a period of stress. It flexes
the spine, aids abdominal muscles and helps to
balance the nervous system. Start from a
kneeling position with both the knees and feet
together and back up straight, arms at sides.
Slowly bend over to curve in a relaxed position
trying to bring the head down to the ground
and as close to the knees as possible. Arms are
relaxed by thighs. Hold for the count of 50.
Work up to finally staying in the pose for 2
minutes. Blank thoughts, please.

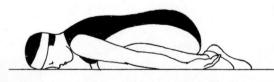

BODY CHECK

Hands are on show all the time — you are frequently judged by the state and expression of your hands. They are a dead give-away of age. Can you show your hands with confidence? Are they supple and graceful? Are they smooth? Are nails clean, neat and manicured? Hands need constant checking. Check on exercises to make hands more flexible and graceful: clench the fist tightly, thumb buried under fingers; open the hand, throwing the fingers forward and spreading wide; hold rigid for a minute; exercise both hands together — clench and open 6 times. Check on the following: do you wear rubber gloves for all wet work? Do you wear heavy gloves for gardening, fabric gloves for housework? Do you wear gloves outdoors when it's cold, raining or snowing? Do you dry your hands well after each washing and then smooth on a hand lotion? Do you scrub fingers and nails daily with a firm brush? Prevention is the best path to beautiful hands, but if your hands are unsightly rub with a pumice stone to remove stains and rough skin. A lemon will clean and bleach fingers. At night rub in vaseline or a heavy handcream, wear gloves. If your hands are dry, the best bath for them is a soak in warm olive oil. Nicotine stains? The most reliable stain removers are peroxide or lemon juice — but then you shouldn't be smoking anyway, should you?

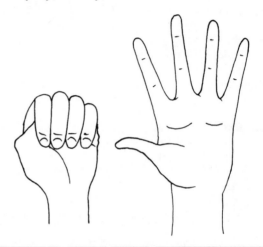

BEAUTY POINTER

You now have your complete make-up range and kit. What do you do? You do your first complete make-over, slowly following the step-by-step guide on the 'Skincare Chart'. Warning: it's not going to work out right this first time. Think of it as a practice trip. After all you are probably using new preparations and for the first time applying new techniques. Be very aware of the contours of your face; emphasize good points with lighter shades, shade away areas you want to diminish. Use your brushes, you'll find it difficult to control them at first, to judge lines, to balance pressure. Practice makes perfect, and remember that any successful make-up depends on 3 things: cosmetics that suit your colouring and personality, the right tools and a confident hand. From now on follow this guide every day.

OPTIONAL

Haven't you always wanted to treat yourself to a whole new range of coordinated skincare preparations. The psychological benefit is as significant as the physical one. And after spending a certain sum you are more inclined to religiously follow a daily routine. Go and inspect the various collections, collect the literature, study it — look into the value of special formula creams and lotions, into potions for wrinkles, firmers for faces. Don't be afraid to ask the skin consultants many questions. Hopefully they can give the right answers, but it's up to you to make the final analysis. And, of course, you can really only judge by trial. It's a luxury that could be an investment for good skin in the future.

DIET

Breakfast:
½ grapefruit
1 boiled egg
1 slice whole-grain toast
coffee or tea

Lunch:
2 slices roast chicken, no skin
1 cup broccoli
1 raw tomato
coffee or tea

Dinner:
175g (6 oz) roast beef or lean steak
1 cup brussels sprouts or spring greens
1 raw tomato
1 apple
coffee or tea

What part do minerals play in nutrition? Do you need to check on whether you are getting enough? The body does indeed need minerals but in very minute quantities. They are essential for certain functions, acting as a catalyst and leave the body through sweat or urine without actually being used up themselves. Do not take mineral supplements in capsule form unless prescribed by your doctor. Amounts required are so tiny, and the dividing line between the required amount and an overdose is very fine. Fresh everyday vegetables provide all we need.

SKIN CARE

Wear no make-up today. Do your cleanse/tone moisturize routine in the morning, then giv yourself a steam facial. Steam encourages the pores to push out dirt and impurities. I promotes perspiration and stimulates circu lation. Steaming with a herb infusion is the most beneficial method. Use camomile, rose mary or thyme — put a handful of the herb in bowl, pour over boiling water, tightly cover fo 3 minutes. Make a towel into a tent, uncove the bowl and steam face for 10 minutes. Blo dry — and that means blot, not rub — apply toner, then moisturize.

BEAUTY POINTER

Today you have time to give yourself a leisurely manicure — and this isn't just a cosmetic treatment for nails, it also conditions both hand and nails and protects them from daily wea and tear. Get your tools together, you'll need small towel, absorbent cotton, nail brush, dish of soapy water, emery board, orange sticks, nai buffer, cuticle cream, handcream, polish re mover, basecoat and nail enamel. It's also good idea to have a basket to put them all in — to keep them tidy and together for future use Now follow the step-by-step manicure procedure illustrated on page 82.

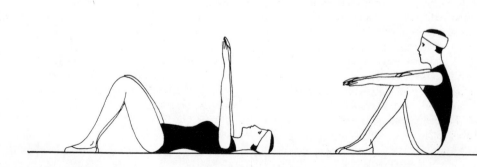

EXERCISE

Despite the fact that this is rest-and-pamper day, don't skip the walk or avoid the exercises. However, whilst taking that extra time in bed, you can do 2 exercises to keep up the good work on legs and stomach. Lazy leg lift: lie on the bed, on your back, arms at sides, palms down; bend right leg, hold to the count of 3; stretch and push to ceiling, count 3; slowly lower to bed. Repeat 6 times; do the same with the left leg. Stomach pull: lie on back, knees bent, feet flat, arms out in front and a little apart. Pull up the torso, so chest touches thighs; lower slowly. Repeat 10 times.

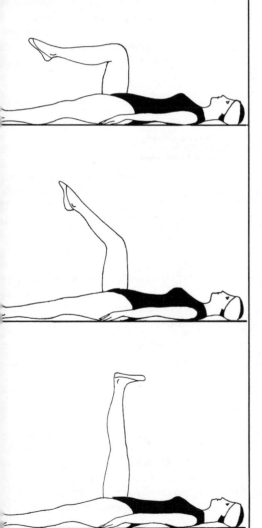

BODY CHECK

Nails. Do you know that nails are horny extensions of the skin? How strong or brittle your nails are is partly a matter of inheritance, but nutrition and care are also of tremendous importance. Nails are good indicators of circulation. Put pressure on the nail, release it and watch how quickly the blood returns. Nails grow at the rate of 6.5 millimetres (¼ inch) a month, so if you start paying attention to them now, you can soon see the results. Look at your nails. What needs attention? Are there ruts, bumps or marks? Horizontal lines mean they've been badly treated at some point, probably an injury to the cuticle, but good care will rectify this. Vertical lines tend to be hereditary and the older you get the more they show. White spots can be a sign of disease or stress or caused by air pockets — they should grow out. Do you take care of your nails properly? Don't put them too much in soap and water — they'll get soft. Don't expose them to extreme cold — they'll get brittle. Don't use a metal nail file — it encourages splitting. Don't cut with scissors or clippers, it will cause splits. Things to do are: shape nails with an emery board and shape them to an oval . . . keep cuticles soft by keeping them well moisturized and push back softened cuticles with a tissue . . . if nails are dry soak them for 5 minutes in warm oil . . . if nails are weak help to strengthen them by directly applying apple cider vinegar or brushing with white iodine.

OPTIONAL

The ultimate luxury is to be able to stay in bed most of the day — to lie and rest, to sip herbal tea, to take a long, leisurely conditioning bath, to do absolutely nothing except relax and read — once you've done everything on this page that is!

DIET

Breakfast:
½ grapefruit
toasted cheese on 1 slice whole-grain toast
coffee or tea

Lunch:
2 slices cold lean beef
1 tomato
8 slices cucumber
1 slice whole-grain toast
1 apple
coffee or tea

Dinner:
125g (4 oz) grilled fish, a smudge of margarine
1 bowl green salad dressed with lemon juice
 and a drop of olive oil
1 sliced orange
coffee or tea

Watch out for complacency! Having stood the course for a week, after losing some weight and beginning to feel and look sleeker, there's a terrible tendency to start to cheat. A bit of sugar here, a drink there, a bigger portion than is indicated. Don't. Be strong. The diet this week is similar to the previous 7 days, but you'll start making things tastier by using herbs and adding juice drinks. So don't cheat. At this point it's not worth it.

BODY CHECK

Special focus on the state of the skin all over: first thing is to get rid of all the flaky dead surface cells. Remember how you treated your face with salt on the first day? Now do the same to the entire body. Wet a flannel, spray with fine kitchen salt and gently rub into the skin. You will need to re-wet the flannel and refurbish the salt several times before the whole body has been rubbed down. Rinse away all salt under a cool shower. Moisturize the skin with body lotion. If you have time, take a nourishing bath after the shower — stir ½kg (1 lb) of oatmeal into a deep warm bath. Relax, soak. Afterwards rinse well with cool water, pat dry and smooth in body lotion.

EXERCISE

Are you used to walking now? This week step up the distance and the time. Walk more briskly and aim for 3.5 kilometres (2 miles) in 35 minutes. It's not that much more than before but it means you are building up stamina. Your daily body work-out also changes, offering slightly more strenuous routines. Follow the 'Second Week Exercise Plan' on page 68. Of course, if you're particularly keen, you can extend your exercise time to 40 minutes and do both routines.

OPTIONAL

Professional attention to nails is bliss — and from a practical point of view, it is the best way to get yourself going on a home-care plan — you'll learn a few tricks too. So if you're having problems with your manicure and simply can't cope with your feet — many women can't even reach them — then off you go to see how the experts do it. Many hairdressing salons and all specialist beauty places offer this service. Don't be shy about nails being in bad condition, after all the manicurist is there to improve them and during the course of her working day she sees many nails in battered condition. But don't be surprised if she raises her eyebrows a bit!

BEAUTY POINTER

Having checked on the state of your feet and started paying more attention to them — hopefully — now pretty them up and give yourself a pedicure. It takes about 20 minutes and it will be awkward at first, but as with everything else, skill comes with practice. You should have a pedicure every 2 or 3 weeks, more often in the summer when you wear open shoes. Assemble your tools. Basically they are the same as for a manicure, but with a few extra items: towel, absorbent cotton, nail brush, pumice stone, large bowl of soapy water, emery board, nail clippers or curved manicure scissors, orange sticks, nail butter, cuticle cream, handcream, nail polish remover, basecoat and nail enamel. Follow the step-by-step procedure illustrated on page 84.

SKIN CARE

As usual cleanse/tone/moisturize. Make your own toner and see how it compares with the commercial product: combine 1 cup of rose water with ½ cup witch hazel; pour into a bottle and shake. That's all. On to another matter: in addition to surface care, facial skin requires a firm support to look smooth and supple. This is provided by muscles, though you may never think of your face as having any. They are no different than any others — and they need to be exercised to keep in condition. Laughter does it, so do these grimaces — do them in front of the mirror. 1. Fill cheeks with air and purse lips. Place 3 fingers of each hand on each cheek. Press fingers against blown-out areas, but don't let air out. Count to 10. Relax. Repeat 5 times. 2. Open mouth wide as if screaming, open eyes wide and stare. Count to 3. Relax. Repeat 5 times. 3. Open mouth wide, fling head back; open and close mouth 5 times. Relax. 4. Purse lips and move mouth from left to right 10 times, then end with a big grin, hold to the count of 5 Relax.

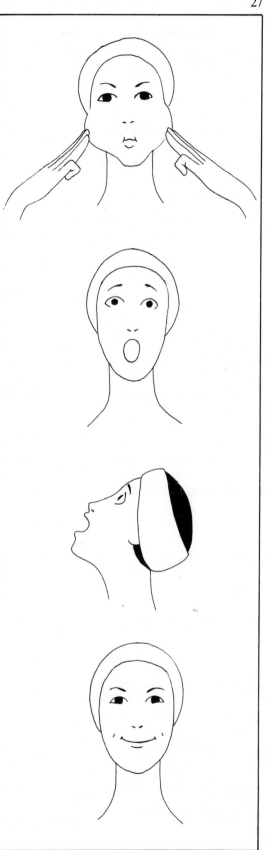

BODY CHECK

Have you ever had thoughts about massage — except that you possibly couldn't afford it, and where would you find a masseur anyway? Wait a minute. Think a bit about its value — it relaxes, it helps circulation, it exercises the skin. You can actually do it to yourself as it's not that difficult to learn the basic techniques. Of course, you cannot massage your back or your buttocks, but everywhere else is within reach. Learn these strokes, these directions of movement and use them when applying body lotion — in this way you are achieving two goals with one effort.

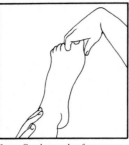

feet: firmly stroke from toes to ankles, one hand on either side of foot. Make a fist with one hand and move knuckles in circular movements over soles. Toe by toe, rotate then pull.

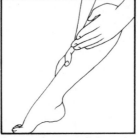

legs: stroke upwards from the ankle, using palms of hands and with more pressure on calf. At knees do circular movements with thumbs over the cap and at sides where fatty deposits are common.

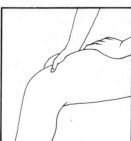

thighs: stroke up the thigh; then working from the knee up, knead and wring the flesh, always pushing upward and towards the centre.

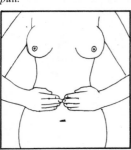

stomach: using palms, stroke in circular movements working towards the centre; increase pressure at the sides and around the waist; finally push upwards over the ribs.

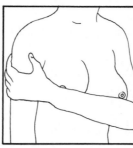

arms: stroke upwards, use circles around the elbow and knead the upper arm using a firm hand clasp.

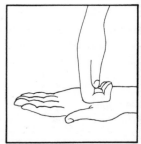

hands: stroke away from fingertips, rotate each finger in turn, then pull; knead the palm with knuckles of clenched fist.

EXERCISE

Check on what you are now doing. The daily walk and exercises? Yes, of course. But what about the other suggestions — having a go one day and forgetting them the next is not good enough. Are you doing the breathing exercise? Before the work-out is the best time. Checked on posture recently? And what about those special movements for legs, feet and hands? Look back and run through them again. And, out of doors — done any cycling lately?

SKIN CARE

Some people sweat more than others, many are embarrassed about it. Do you have this problem? The reason for sweating is to put water on your skin where it cools it through evaporation. Sweat itself does not smell, odour is caused by bacteria that get trapped in airless areas — hairy spots are more prone, most notably under the arms. Are you coping properly with perspiration? Daily bathing deals with general sweating. You can control odour under the arms by using a deodorant — it is helpful if you remove underarm hair by shaving. A deodorant is a chemical compound which hinders the bacterial action. One application a day is usually sufficient — but apply to a clean area. An anti-perspirant has an additional asset — it limits wetness as well as coping with bacteria. It contains more chemicals and can be irritating. A do-it-yourself method works well: put ½ cup of cider vinegar in 1 cup distilled water. Keep in an airtight bottle, shake before use. Apply to underarm area with cotton pads. The smell of vinegar disappears in about 15 minutes — so there's no need to worry about that!

BEAUTY POINTER

What happened to your hair last week? Are you happy with it? Judge by these guidelines: Is the style right for your face? Is it right for your lifestyle? Can you easily cope with it yourself — brush or comb it into place, control it with a blow dryer or hot curlers? Did it more or less stay in good shape all week — or did it fall apart the following day? Is the colour right? Did it become very dry? Did you have to wash it within a few days because it was greasy? If you're satisfied it is just fine, then start to take care of it yourself — remembering to go and have it cut if necessary about every 6 to 8 weeks. If you're not content, go back to the same hairstylist and explain why. Let the same person have another go. Don't change hairdressers immediately — though you may have to eventually. It is often difficult to do hair correctly the first time — a stylist has to get to know texture, condition and reaction to preparations.

DIET

Breakfast:
½ grapefruit
1 boiled egg
1 slice whole-grain toast
coffee or tea

Lunch:
fruit salad — 1 orange, 1 apple, 1 slice
    pineapple or melon, 1 banana, a few grapes
    plus the juice of a lemon
2 tablespoons cottage cheese
coffee or tea

Dinner:
2 slices lean lamb, no skin
1 cup brussels sprouts or broccoli
1 tomato
1 slice whole-grain toast
coffee or tea

When eating less than usual, the worst time of day is often just before going to bed — particularly if you've been used to having a nibble at that time or a substantial hot drink. This may mean you are having trouble getting to sleep. In addition, less food intake can make the mind more active and sleep may not come easily. A calming, soothing drink at bedtime is camomile tea (see page 34); better still — but more difficult to find — is valerian; look for it at a herbalist or health food store.

OPTIONAL

Do you ever seek the unusual in health and beauty care? One of the most intriguing theories is that essences of flowers can help both physical and emotional states. Healing by means of aromatic essences is an ancient art, but it was an English physician Dr Edward Bach who pioneered a new way of flower power during the 1920s. His theory stated that the mental outlook of a patient is the guide to which remedy to use. The flower potions, harmless in themselves, are capable of conveying a forceful energy pattern which is often the key to natural cures. For example, gentian is said to help self doubt and depression, rock rose is for panic. There are over 30 remedies available at specialist chemists. Seek them out.

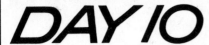

DIET

Breakfast:
1 slice melon
1 sliced orange
1 slice whole-grain toast
coffee or tea

Lunch:
125g (4 oz) grilled fish
green salad with lemon juice
½ grapefruit
coffee or tea

Dinner:
2 slices lean beef
2 sticks celery braised with a little margarine
1 tomato
6 slices cucumber
½ grapefruit
coffee or tea

Has your weight not moved for 2 days? This can often happen after 8 or 9 days of a diet. Body weight reaches a certain plateau and seems disinclined to budge. Don't worry. If you are following the diet exactly, pounds will begin to shift again. Meanwhile if you want to give your body a push — and if you can bear it — just eat apples today instead of the set menus, but don't eat more than 8.

SKIN CARE

You've been giving your face a fair amount of daily attention. Has its condition improved? Is there anything that is bothering you? Conditions such as dryness, areas of oil, flaky surfaces should now be well under control. Maybe you have red pimples or spots. There are inflammations of the skin and little can be done to prevent them as they are either hereditary or caused by hormone changes. Never squeeze them unless a blackhead or pus is there — if you do the spot will get bigger and harder. Wait until pus develops, then gently let it out. Blackheads are the most common form of blemish — you can squeeze them yourself, but hygiene is imperative. Whiteheads are more difficult as these are tiny white beads of waxy matter under the skin and have no way out to the surface unless helped by breaking the skin. A tiny opening has to be made — it is best done by a skin specialist. Spider veins need professional care if they really bother you, but most are easily concealed by make-up. If skin blemishes are bad to the point of being acne, make an appointment with a dermatologist at once. Don't mess around on your own even with medication from a chemist. Today nearly all cases of acne are curable with the right care.

BEAUTY POINTER

You're on your own with your hair today. If you are pleased with your new cut, new image, check that you know how to take care of it correctly. There are 4 steps to good hair: shampooing, rinsing, conditioning, drying. Refer to page 92 for all the details. Don't just go ahead, none of the procedures are as straightforward as you may think — and you'll be surprised how many women even wash their hair incorrectly. So check. Then you need to consider special rinses and conditioning creams. Can you cope with colour on your own? What about problems like dandruff? Do you need to set your hair? Blow it dry? Do you know how? All guidelines are on pages 92 to 96.

BODY CHECK

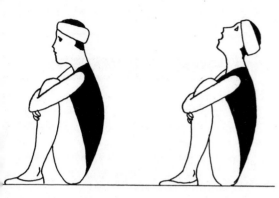

Neck check: it is so easy to forget this area, but what a barometer of ageing and neglect it is! Bad muscle habits in the neck cause crepiness and lines. The neck is not an isolated section of the body, but part of good posture which contributes greatly to keeping the throat smooth and agile. Try this exercise: sit with knees up to chest, head inclined forward; pull neck up, shoulders down; slowly pull the head back as far as possible, open and close mouth 3 times. Return to forward relaxed position. Repeat 5 times. Throats can get very dry — don't forget to moisturize when doing facial routine. If necessary, use a special throat cream during the night.

EXERCISE

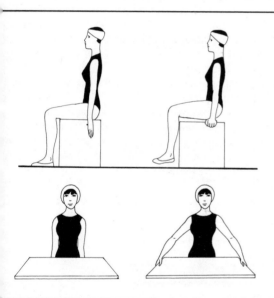

Are you an office worker, having to fit your daily walk and exercises into precious leisure hours? Well, there are 2 easy yet constructive movements you can do sitting at your desk. They follow the isometric principle of setting muscle strength against that of an immobile force. 1. Sit on chair, arms at sides; place palms on chair and lift buttocks and thighs off the chair, feet off the floor; hold steady to the count of 6. Lower body, relax. Repeat 10 times — or as often as you can during the day. 2. Sit in front of the desk, arms at sides; raise arms and clutch edges of table; push hard as though squeezing the table, count to 6. Relax. Repeat 10 times — or whenever.

OPTIONAL

Indulge in a day of beauty. Many salons, clubs and health farms offer a day-long programme for a special price. This usually includes a sauna, swim, exercise, massage, maybe a special skin treatment such as a wax bath. You'll be given a facial, maybe a manicure and pedicure. Hair will be done and face made up if you like.

You'll have time to rest, have a snooze; you'll eat light, healthy food — and go home feeling on top of the world. Make enquiries today and arrange for such a day, maybe for after the 21-day regime, to give you a lift and an extra incentive to continue taking care of your body and beauty in the most constructive way.

DIET

Breakfast:
½ grapefruit
1 boiled egg
1 slice whole-grain toast
coffee or tea

Lunch:
2 tablespoons cottage cheese
1 tomato
1 cup sliced boiled courgettes
1 slice whole-grain toast
coffee or tea

Dinner:
3 slices boiled or roasted chicken, no skin
1 cup coarsely chopped spinach
1 cup string beans
1 apple
coffee or tea

Food so far has been very plain. There's been a reason for this — to get you completely away from sauces, from frying, from butter and cream. But now think about herbs as flavouring. You can add them to any of the menus — it's already been suggested to add tarragon to fish. Herbs will give a lift to the basic foods, encourage you to continue now that a new taste is added. Some ideas: basil — good with fish, egg and tomato dishes; dill — with fish, salads, vegetables; marjoram — lamb; rosemary — chicken; sage — fish and egg dishes.

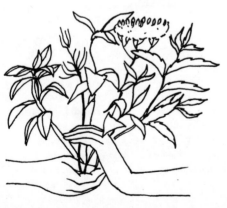

BEAUTY POINTER

You did your first new step-by-step make-up last week. You've now had 5 days to get more skilful, to experiment. Now that you have a general view of your new face, you must examine each step, analyse it and be sure you have it right. First check on your foundation. Happy with the colour? Put your day face under scrutiny (evening tactics are discussed later). Do you make-up in direct light? If you are still not doing so, make a point of it today. Now what about faults, are you covering them up in the best way? Do you know how to camouflage a pimple, narrow a nose, detract from a heavy jaw, disguise a late night? Refer to make-up tips on the Skincare Chart. Study the foundation section and get it all right. Remember most important is to blend in the shades so no-one can tell where one ends and the other begins — otherwise you can look like a jigsaw puzzle. Correct shading gives a face its undulations, and undulations give a face its character and beauty. So work at it. Today, devote time to your foundation technique — become an artist.

SKIN CARE

Preparations you make at home can be as effective as a commercial product. Sometimes claims go a bit over the top, particularly from the nature-is-everything brigade. But don't dismiss them because they appear so simple. Make and try this skin-firming lotion. They've been good reports about it. Use it today in place of your normal toner. If you like it, continue using it twice a day for 3 days. The recipe is: 1 tablespoon fresh cucumber juice (obtained through a juice extractor or a sieve), 3 tablespoons rose water, 1 teaspoon benzoin (from a chemist). Mix all ingredients together, keep in a cool place. Apply with a cotton wad.

EXERCISE

Are you managing to cover that mileage on foot every day? And don't you dare admit you're not doing the daily exercises. Add a bit of fun today: skip. Yes, just that. Get hold of a child's skipping rope and do it indoors or out. Believe it or not, this is marvellous exercise for the whole body. Start skipping slowly and work up to 100 jumps a minute — well try anyway. Skip barefoot or in gym shoes.

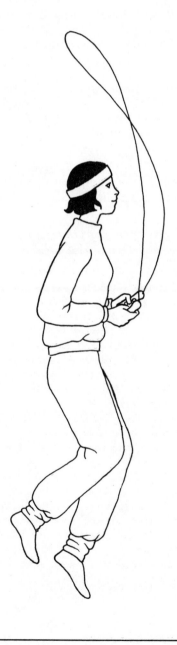

BODY CHECK

Sleep — are you getting enough of it? What is enough for that matter? The old rule was 8 hours, but now that is considered to be just the average because recent research shows that some people need as few as 5 hours and others have to snooze away for 11. Only you can judge how much you need. Do you wake up feeling refreshed or lousy? Can you get through the day without feeling whacked? Do you often think: I simply have to get more sleep? It's up to you. It appears there's a lot to be said for the old rule of 'early to bed and early to rise etc.' Sleep is essential for mental and physical health — it recharges energy, puts the psyche in order, restores capabilities, refreshes the brain and balances metabolism. You only have to be without it for some time to realize all of this is true. If you're not sleeping well, or have difficulty getting to sleep, make a note of these points: go to bed when you are tired, don't rigidly stick to a certain bedtime; sleep in a cool room but a warm bed; take a relaxing bath before going to bed, add a few drops of orange blossom essence to the bath; a herb pillow often helps sleep, make it of hops and lime blossom; a comfortable bed, fresh sheets and a pretty bedroom make all the difference . . . and shut out any noise.

OPTIONAL

Who hasn't wanted to be made-up by an expert? What tricks can you learn? What face can you have? Taking a make-up lesson from a professional is an optional that is a curious mixture of plus and minus. Of course, it depends who does it. Make-up artists are expert at skill, but not always expert at judging your face, your personality, your individual style. You can come out looking marvellous, but you can also come out looking like a painted doll and not you at all. What you can learn is how to use cosmetics. You can see — and will be shown — how to put on everything, the best way to use pencils and brushes, where to shade, where to blush etc. It is interesting to go and see how someone else looks at your face — you can possibly strike a balance between that idea and yours. And you've had a first hand view of how to do it.

DIET

Breakfast:
½ grapefruit
toasted cheese on 1 slice whole-grain bread
coffee or tea

Lunch:
2 tablespoons cottage cheese
2 cups raw spinach, coarsely chopped,
  seasoned with lemon and 1 teaspoon olive
  oil
1 slice whole-grain toast
coffee or tea

Dinner:
125g (4 oz) fillet grilled fish
1 bowl green salad
1 slice whole-grain toast
coffee or tea

During this regime camomile has often been mentioned. Do you know that it is one of the oldest recognized herbs and a favourite with herbalists for generations? It is an acquired taste, but acquire it if you can because taken daily it contributes to general well-being. Tea bags are available, but you can also make your own infusion (it's better to do so). Take 25g (1 oz) flowers to 575ml (1 pint) boiling water. Cover and allow to steep for 5 minutes. This drink is excellent for nervous conditions, it also helps indigestion, relieves stomach pain, is good for premenstrual cramps and is an aid for the kidneys. It can make you calm for sleep. Try and see what it can do for you. Get some camomile today.

OPTIONAL

If you enjoyed the massage last week, you should have made an appointment for today. If you are going to consider massage as part of your beauty programme it should be done on a regular weekly basis — the odd massage here and there isn't of any prolonged benefit. Maybe you'd like to take your own cream or perfumed oil today. And having had one massage, you'll return better equipped to judge the technique, the value — do you think it strong enough, do you completely relax, is the tenseness taken away from the back of the neck? Talk to your masseur about your reactions — it's invaluable to you both.

BEAUTY POINTER

Still on make-up . . . well better stick to it until you get it right — then that's one aspect finished and organized. Look at blusher today. And you should look at it well, because it is the ultimate controller of an individual face. It can enliven the face, it can change its shape, it gives colour. It can make or break you — so to speak. Colour is difficult to decide upon. It is not adequate to say it should blend with your skin — which many experts suggest — because it should accentuate your best features and sometimes this can only be done with strong or contrasting colour. Most important is to know where to apply it, how much to use, when to emphasize, when to control. That is where your individuality and sense of panache come into it. You can learn the rules by following the guide on the 'Skincare Chart' but in the long run it is you who decides and determines the effect. Play around with blusher today — try different spots, different strengths. You may grimace at some of the results — but that's good facial exercise after all!

BODY CHECK

When did you last see a doctor? To go for help when you feel ill is one thing, but have you taken any precautionary checks lately? Anticipating what can go wrong is one of the positive things of medicine today. So make an appointment for a general checkup with your GP. Also do you know what your blood group is? You should. Any idea of your blood pressure? Find out. Also as a woman it is of paramount importance that you go and see a gynaecologist once a year. You need to have a pap smear test to detect pre-cancerous states, you need to have a professional breast examination (how to examine your own see page 42). If you have not had these checks for years you are foolish — but you are not the only one, it is a very common fault to ignore preventive measures now available to everyone. Telephone and make appointments.

SKIN CARE

Have you ever considered that your kitchen shelf can provide many worthwhile ingredients to help your skin? You've learnt about salt to take away dead cells, about oatmeal for a nourishing bath, about olive oil for dryness, about lemon for cleansing. Here are some other things to check on: cider vinegar — as a toner, put 1 teaspoon in 1½ cups distilled water; honey — as a conditioner, massage it raw into the face, leave on for 20 minutes, rinse away; butter — as an aid to very dry skin, melt a teaspoon and beat in 2 tablespoons milk, apply to face and leave on a few hours; eggs — for a facial that works really well, take an egg yolk, three drops of cider vinegar, a ½ teaspoon of olive oil, mix together and apply to the skin for 10 minutes, rinse away; powdered milk — for a modern version of the ancient milk bath, put 1 cup in a bath of warm water.

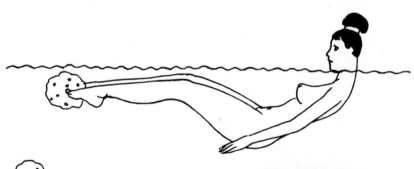

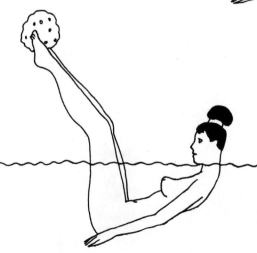

EXERCISE

Just in case you are slacking about your walk and not really putting your heart into that daily dozen, when bathing today make up for it by doing these movements . . . and make a note to do them from this day on. 1. Lie back, grab a sponge or flannel between your feet, slowly raise legs as high as possible, pull in the stomach and hold to the count of 3, lower slowly. Repeat 5 times. 2. Begin with legs straight in front, bend one knee, then push the leg up to the ceiling, stretching the knee and flexing the foot, hold straight to the count of 10, return through bending knee and into the water. Do 5 times with each leg.

DAY 13

SKIN CARE

The skin around the eye is particularly delicate — and particularly prone to lines. Are you in need of special attention here? This area needs a light fingertip touch and often a special cream — the older you are the more necessary. There are some extremely effective commercial eyecreams, and although prices are high, it's definitely worth it. A natural aid is to dot on a few drops of almond oil morning and night. You can also benefit from an all-night treatment of cotton wads soaked in warm almond oil, held in place with a sleeping mask or wide bandage. An emergency cover-up for a special occasion is egg white which will smooth the under-eye area for a few hours. Pat on a very thin film of unbeaten white of an egg, better still brush it on with a sable brush — the thinner the coating, the more effective; allow to dry and then apply make-up, but pat on with fingertips instead of smoothing in.

EXERCISE

By now you should be getting considerably fitter and able to manage more complicated body movements. So after your walk and exercises today, see if you can do the Yoga shoulder stand. It's a very valuable posture as it reverses the flow of blood and stimulates the endocrine system, plus stretching practically every muscle of the body. Start by lying flat on your back, legs outstretched, arms parallel to the body, palms down. Raise the legs slowly, keeping the knees straight and tightly together, toes pointing. Continue until legs are about a third of the way to a vertical position; pause. By pressing hands and elbows on the floor try to elevate legs until vertical, then lift the hips, back and stomach and finally chest, sliding hands under the small of the back to support and balance the torso. Hold for a few minutes, slowly return by first bending the knees then lowering the torso and finally straightening the legs. If you practise this, in time you should be able to hold the body vertical for several minutes. It's terribly good for you. And it gives you another eye view of the world.

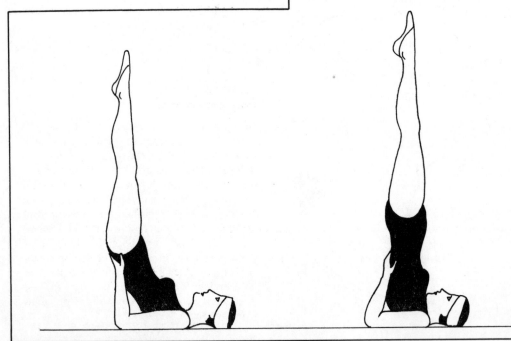

DIET

Breakfast:
1 slice melon
50g (2 oz) poached fillet of fish
1 slice whole-grain toast
coffee or tea

Lunch:
1 large bowl fruit salad with lemon juice
coffee or tea

Dinner:
2 slices cold chicken or turkey, no skin
1 tomato
½ bunch watercress
1 slice whole-grain toast
coffee or tea

Do you normally use garlic when you cook? If you don't, you should and you can now start adding it to this diet — just a little finely chopped raw garlic to provide extra flavour to salads and vegetables. Don't worry, you are not going to reek of it, and in any case its smell can be counteracted by chewing a spring of fresh parsley. Garlic has become synonymous with health, energy and longevity for good reason. Try this garlic tonic: mince 2 garlic cloves and steep in a glass of dry white wine for 3 days; take a teaspoon first thing every morning.

OPTIONAL

All right, so you're not entirely convinced that neutral shades are the best for eyes, and you'd really like to prove your point by experimenting with more colours. There's nothing to stop you going out and buying every shade you can — but look for a paintbox of eye colours. That's an optional that's not such a luxury because for a reasonable cost you can get a whole range of possibilities to play around with. What is a luxury is the time! Time to experiment, time to play around with 20 or more shades.

BEAUTY POINTER

Eyes give your face its expression and most women like to emphasize eyes above all other features. Rightly so. Do you know how to make-up your eyes superbly? There are techniques for all shapes of eyes (see Skincare Chart) which means that any eye can emerge as a striking feature. The best results can be achieved with just a combination of eye-crayon and shadow. If you learn to blend these properly, that's all you need. Neutral smoky colours — the greys and the browns — are the most natural and can be the most effective. It's so easy to go wrong with bright colours. Then you'll need mascara and an eyebrow pencil. Again to repeat what's been said before — it's not the range of products that matter, but the skill. Use brushes, use applicators and follow the chart. Sooner or later you'll get your eye right.

BODY CHECK

More focus on eyes. First, can you focus properly? When did you last have your eyes checked? Even if your vision is perfect, there's the possibility of some ailment, such as glaucoma, lurking there and if caught early can be quickly and efficiently dealt with. So if you haven't seen an optologist for ages, if ever, make an appointment. What's wrong with your eyes that *you* can cope with? Bloodshot? Commercial drops help but it's bad to use them constantly. Try compresses of camomile infusion or simply put cooled-down camomile teabags on each eye. Puffy? One of the best things is a slice of raw potato under each eye, or better still if you have the time, grate a raw potato and put a teaspoonful or two on muslin squares to cover both the lid and the under-eye area of closed eye. Leave on for 15 minutes, then splash with cold water. Tired looking? Soak cotton pads in witch hazel, close eyelids, place pads over them and lie down for half an hour — be careful not to let the liquid enter the eyes — it stings and makes them bloodshot.

DAY 14

DIET

Breakfast:
1 large bowl fresh fruit salad
any type of tea

Lunch:
1 large bowl vegetable soup
  (to be made exactly as recipe on page 60)
any type of tea

Dinner:
1 large bowl vegetable soup
any type of tea

The diet takes a different path today and for the next 3 days — it's a fruit and vegetable regime only. This is a way of making sure that the body is well cleared of toxic matter and also helps to bring down weight level. It is something that is frequently done at health farms. It is important to follow exactly as stated and don't eat fruit at any other meal except breakfast. You'll find it more substantial than it appears.

SKIN CARE

Exfoliate facial skin with salt, rinse many times with cool water and then give yourself a conditioning facial. There are many commercial masks to choose from. They act as cleansers and purifiers. All rely on a drying process and they are rinsed or peeled off. Two good ones you can make yourself: 1 teaspoon of powdered yeast mixed with 2 teaspoons warm water; add more water if it doesn't spread on like paste. Or combine 2 tablespoons honey and ½ teaspoon of lemon juice or cider vinegar — this is particularly good for dry skins. Procedure: start with a clean face, smooth hair away; apply mask all over face and throat; leave free circles over eye areas and cover them with cottonwool pads soaked in milk or witch hazel. Keep eyes closed; lie down and relax for 20 minutes. Look out for any special instructions if you use a commercial preparation. Remove all traces of mask, rinse well, blot dry, apply moisturizer — and don't wear make-up for the rest of the day.

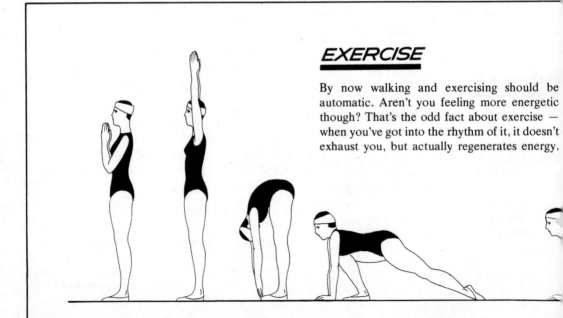

EXERCISE

By now walking and exercising should be automatic. Aren't you feeling more energetic though? That's the odd fact about exercise — when you've got into the rhythm of it, it doesn't exhaust you, but actually regenerates energy.

BEAUTY POINTER

Manicure day, same procedure as last week (see page 82). If you notice your nails are dry, soak in warm olive oil for 10 minutes — but you need to scrub them with soap and water afterwards otherwise polish will not adhere. As you're not wearing any make-up today it's a good time to play around with lip techniques. Put a little foundation base on the lips and consult the make-up guide on the Skincare Chart. The most effective way is to use a crayon to outline the lips and a brush for filling in. Watch shape, watch colour. Lipstick shades can be tricky as they often change colour once on the lips due to personal skin chemistry. You can re-contour the mouth within limits — learn the shading tricks, draw different shapes. Caution: don't go overboard on change. Concentrate on finding the right mouth while your face is clear of other make-up distractions.

BODY CHECK

Bad breath a problem? It's something you have to check on yourself, because it's rare someone else would have the nerve to mention it. It's caused by something decomposing in the mouth, not necessarily food particles but also because of gum disease. It can invariably be prevented by good oral hygiene. The juice of any green vegetable is a natural antidote because of the high percentage of chlorophyll. Don't overuse commercial mouthwashes, particularly those that claim to freshen breath — they can upset the mouth's natural flora balance. Hydrogen peroxide can be used regularly; this kills bacteria and strengthens gums. Try a natural mouthwash: cold peppermint tea, or a mixture of equal proportions of rosemary and mint steeped in water for 30 minutes; strain before use.

OPTIONAL

Pampering day — get as much rest as possible. Catch up on the newest magazines. Spend time on yourself, the one day you really can. If it's a lovely day, go for a longer walk than usual, not so briskly, but a leisurely hour or so in the fresh air. Persuade someone to learn those massage strokes (see page 28) and end the day with an indulgent relaxing massage with soft music in the background. It's all very therapeutic.

Hopefully you are greeting the day with renewed enthusiasm — to make early moments more rewarding try this sequence of movements based on Yoga principles. It's the best way to the first deep breath of the day, the first big stretch. Do it 3 times — and first thing in the morning from now on: stand straight, feet lightly apart, hands in prayer position; lift arms over head, then bend over and try to touch toes; using hands to support body, bend left knee and push right leg back as far as possible, now bring left leg to join the right one; pushing bottom up, lower stomach, push legs back until flat on floor; arch torso and throw back the head; hold for a minute; relax. This exercise is a continuous one; all positions should glide into each other and breathing should be regular and even.

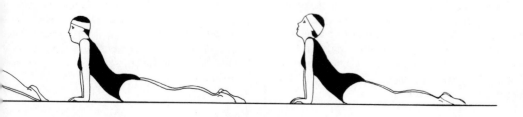

DAY 15

● On the last lap

DIET

Breakfast:
1 large bowl fresh fruit salad
any type of tea

Lunch:
1 large bowl vegetable soup
(to be made exactly as recipe on page 60)
any type of tea

Dinner:
1 large bowl vegetable soup
any type of tea

Continue with the fruit and vegetable plan, but if you like you may have this spiced tomato drink at mid-morning or afternoon: 1 cup tomato juice, 4 tablespoons brewer's (powdered) yeast, 1 tablespoon chopped parsley, ½ table-spoon chopped chives. Mix together, add the merest pinch of salt, lots of ground pepper; refrigerate before drinking.

BEAUTY POINTER

Today's goal: the 7-minute face. If you've been making up your face following the step-by-step guide on the Skincare Chart, you should be pretty efficient by now. But how long does it take you? A daytime make-up (more on an evening face tomorrow) should take no more than 7 minutes. Time yourself. If you're slower, work out what's taking up too much time. Maybe you're putting on too much make-up, emphasizing too many things. Check it all out. Is it natural looking? A good make-up shouldn't look as though it's been plotted and planned, nor should it look as though it's taken hours to apply. So watch that time — it could be better spent doing something else.

EXERCISE

A change of exercises again. This is the fina stage. Use the 'New You Exercise Plan' whicl comes as a chart (loose with the book). Th routines are more demanding than last week and formulate your daily fitness programme fo after the 21-day regime is over. Get them righ this week and continue thereafter in order t maintain your present level, indeed improv your figure further. Walk as usual, do the earl morning Yoga stretches, check that breathin exercise.

OPTIONAL

Have you heard about aromatherapy? It come under the category of alternative medicine bu is also significant in beauty therapy. Th underlying principle is that aromatic essentia oils (those from plants) can help cure b restoring the natural rhythm of the body. Th oils are massaged into the skin, particularly int the main nerve points down the length of th spine. It offers probably the most beneficial o all massages — certainly the most euphoric Seek out an aromatherapist and see for yoursel The body benefits, the skin and the senses. An it's not just because of the massage, th absorption of oil, the manipulations. Of rea importance is the effect of the fragrances o the psychic and mental state. Scents can caus a state of relaxation, relieving tension and inne traumas. On the other hand, powers o perception can become clearer and more acute It depends on the oils, the art and judgement o the therapist. A treatment lasts about an hou and understandably a series is more beneficia than just one.

BODY CHECK

Can you give a dazzling smile with confidence that your teeth are perfect? Have you been to the dentist for a check and clean within the last 6 months? If not, make an appointment right now. Most important, are you cleaning them properly? That means more than brushing. Most cavities start between teeth and in order to remove plaque you need to use dental floss as well. Check on your teeth tactics: clean a minimum of twice a day, morning and evening. Place brush again outside surface at a 45° angle. Move it back and forth with short strokes, sliding bristles so they splay along the gum line. Brush all surfaces this way. Now brush top teeth both inside and out from the gum downwards, then bottom teeth from gum line upwards. Finally use the dental floss. Take about 45cm (18 inches) and wrap ends around middle fingers, leaving a free section of about 2.5cm (1 inch) in the middle. With a slow sawing motion, coax the floss between teeth, slide it a little way into the gum crevice. Pull the floss back and forth. Don't hurt the gums, though most likely they will bleed if you've never flossed before — as gums get healthier and stronger this will stop. You must take the floss between each tooth, making your way around the entire mouth. This is the only way to remove plaque and bacteria thoroughly — and prevent gum disease. Make a note to do it from this day on.

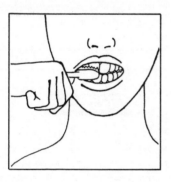
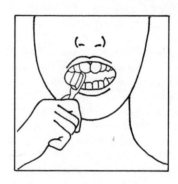
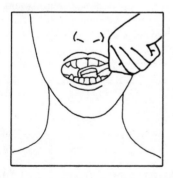
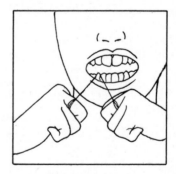

SKIN CARE

Your lips have skin too and are invariably more affected by wind, cold and sun than the rest of the face. Are yours dry? Inclined to get chapped? The first area to blister? Lips do need protection — lipstick does just this, so if you don't wear any you need to use a greasy lip block or vaseline as a buffer against the elements. You can make your own lip salve: 40g (1½ oz) beeswax, 30g (1 oz) honey, 55g (2 oz) sesame oil; melt the beeswax in a double boiler; blend in honey, then oil and whisk to a smooth consistency.

DAY 16

BODY CHECK

Examine your breasts — this should be done once a month and the best time is just after your period has finished. (Make a note to do it again then.) Important is to get to know your breasts — shape, size, undulations, blemishes — as the whole point of this examination is to detect change. First you must be aware of what is normal for you. Check for lumps (less than 10% are cancerous, but they must be seen by a doctor) . . . check for puckering of the skin . . . for new prominence of veins . . . for inverted nipples . . . for discharge from the nipples . . . for enlarged lymph glands (area at side of breast and under armpit) . . . for any moles or blemishes that seem to be changing shape or colour. If anything seems different, or if in doubt, go to your doctor. In any case, you should have a professional check once a year. Self examination guidelines: 1. Inspect by looking into a mirror, get to know breast shape and characteristics. 2. Stretch arms above head, observe any changes. 3. Place hands on hips, check shape and fall. 4. Lie down and feel each breast in turn, starting at the nipple work outwards in finger-traced circles. 5. Still lying down, with flattened fingers test area at the sides of the breast and well into the armpit.

OPTIONAL

You've learned some elementary Yoga postures and practices so far, and if this makes you curious to study more, look for a Yoga teacher and take regular classes. Yoga positions (asanas) and breathing exercises (pranayama) can be learned and practised at any age, but they do require qualified instruction. Postures are awkward and personal guidance is best so you can get them right from the start. Yoga is one of the most practical ways of counteracting stress and tension.

EXERCISE

Still walking each day? You'd better be. Beginning today improve speed, increase distance. Aim for 4 kilometres (2½ miles) in 45 minutes. And try and do more than the regular 20 minutes of exercise — quickly run through the first week's plan in 10 minutes — they should appear very easy now — and then do the final week's series in 20 minutes.

The Five Step Breast Guide

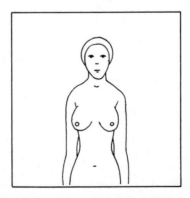
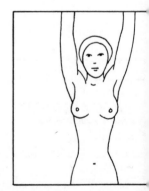

BEAUTY POINTER

Are you using the same make-up for day and evening? You can use the same cosmetics, but you need to intensify the colours, and for extra glamour it's fun to add irridescent highlights and gleam here and there. Light changes colour, affects tone and depth. At night, under artificial light you need emphasis and shine. You need to strengthen both the colour and the line emphasis on the eyes. You need to put on more mascara. Blusher, in particular, must be intensified. Lips need shine — so add a coat of lipgloss or a smear of vaseline. Gold, silver, bronze and irridescent white highlights can brighten and accentuate areas above and around the eyes.

DIET

Breakfast:
1 large bowl fresh fruit salad
any type of tea

Lunch:
1 large bowl vegetable soup
  (to be made exactly as recipe on page 60)

Dinner:
1 large bowl vegetable soup
any type of tea

This is the last day of the fruit and vegetable only regime, so bear with it because tomorrow the diet gets more varied again — and today you can also have the spiced tomato drink of yesterday.

SKIN CARE

Your skin has been getting good basic care during the daily routine of cleanse/tone/ moisturize, plus some special treatments. Does it need any extra attention during the night? Think how it has been reacting over the past 2 weeks. If it is still very dry, it needs an overnight conditioning cream. This should be applied very lightly as the skin can only absorb so much. There are many preparations available, check out the various types and watch the labels (see page 76). You can make your own simple conditioning cream: 400g (14 oz) almond oil, 140g (5 oz) white wax, 1 cup distilled water, few drops spirit vinegar. Melt the oil and wax in a double boiler; drop by drop beat in the combination of water and vinegar. If your skin seems in good condition, or inclined to oiliness, a film of moisturizer is the best nightly care.

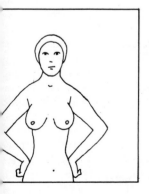
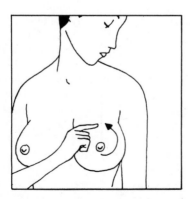
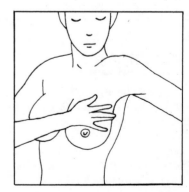

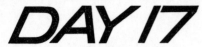

DAY 17

DIET

Breakfast:
½ grapefruit
1 egg scrambled with a smudge of margarine
1 slice whole-grain toast
coffee or tea

Lunch:
125g (4 oz) grilled fish, a little margarine on top
1 bowl green salad
1 slice whole-grain toast
1 orange
coffee or tea

Dinner:
2 grilled lamb chops — cut away all fat
1 cup coarsely chopped cabbage
1 tomato
1 apple
coffee or tea

Remember you can use garlic when you like — for taste and health reasons. You can also have a mid-morning and mid-afternoon juice drink. The best way is to make these is with a juice extractor for the vegetables (or through a sieve) and with a squeezer for the fruit. Raw juices only, nothing boiled. Don't mix fruit and vegetable juices. Choose from: vegetables — beetroot, cabbage, carrot, celery, cucumber, spinach, tomato, watercress; fruits — lemon, orange, grapefruit; apples, apricots and pineapple can be eaten intact.

OPTIONAL

Massage day again. Are you feeling the benefit? If you have time, take a sauna first. Look for a salon that offers the two together, or another complementary body treatment. Some beauticians, give wax baths before a massage. Your body is covered with warm liquid paraffin wax. As it cools and solidifies on your body, it traps in the heat, thus helping to draw out impurities and excess water — and leaves skin very smooth.

EXERCISE

Walk, exercise, get out the bike again — you are meant to be working up to 30 minutes of continuous cycling 3 times a week. Have you got good muscle tone? Improvement so far should be considerable, but for strengthening muscles there's nothing like lifting an extra weight. Won't that build bulky biceps, you may ask? No, because a woman's hormones are a protection, and you are hardly going to dedicate your exercise plan to weight-lifting and body build-up. What you can do is to make your muscles work a little harder, by every 3 or 4 days adding weights to the ankles when doing leg movements. Great for legs and thighs. Use 1.5kg (3 lb) weights; the easiest are weighted plastic strips which tie around the ankle. They can be found in sportshops.

BODY CHECK

Ears: the less you interfere with them the better. More than regular outside cleaning (and a gentle swab with a cotton tip) is not advisable. Poking around to dislodge impacted wax can be harmful. If you think accumulated wax is affecting hearing, go and have ears syringed. This involves jetting water at the eardrum; the wax is pushed out from inside. It's an odd sensation, tickles, but is not painful. Of course any continuing problem with hearing or constant earache needs professional care. Want to have your ears pierced? Many women dither about this, thinking it either hurts or is irreversible. Neither is true. It's done by a gun or needle, so quickly that it's over before you realize it's started. There will be a little discharge at first, and you'll need to wear stud sleepers (best in gold). On the other hand, if you regret your decision immediately, don't put in the sleepers and within a short while the ears will have closed up again. This, however, can only be achieved within a couple of days of having the ears pierced.

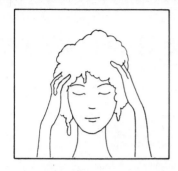

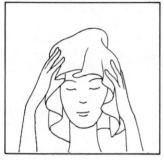

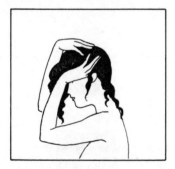

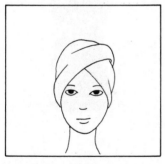

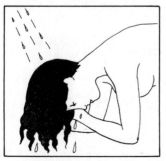

BEAUTY POINTER

Give your hair a deep conditioning treatment. This is quite different from the conditioning application after washing, which is superficial. It is imperative if your hair is dry, and is of considerable benefit for all types of hair. Even if you have your hair regularly taken care of at the hairdresser, you may as well do the home treatment too — it's a less expensive and usually more thorough than those at a salon. Good simple conditioners: for dry, brittle hair — 2 tablespoons of warm olive oil (more if you have lots of hair); for other hair, even oily — beat 2 eggs, continue beating and slowly add 1 tablespoon of olive oil, 1 tablespoon glycerine and 1 teaspoon cider vinegar. Procedure for deep conditioning: 1. Shampoo hair and rinse until clean, till it squeaks. 2. Blot with a towel, comb out tangles. 3. Section hair and rub in conditioner, massage very well into the scalp, make sure conditioner covers all strands. 4. Dip a towel in hot water, wring out, wrap around head and leave on for 30 minutes — to keep towel warm you can cover with a plastic cap. 5. Shampoo lightly, rinse many many times. Allow to dry naturally.

SKIN CARE

Make sure everything is organized for body skincare in the bath. If all your preparations are arranged attractively and in full view of the bath tub, you'll be reminded to use them. Don't tuck them away in a cupboard. Practical basics are: for all skins — salt for the rub down, oatmeal and dried milk for nourishing baths, muslin bags of herbs for a reviving soak (best mix is 1 cup lavender flowers, ½ cup mint leaves, ½ cup rosemary, put into little bags and hang on the hot tap whilst water is running) and a large jar of body lotion. Extras for dry skins — a bath oil, super rich body lotion. Extras for oily skins — a muslin bag of dried or fresh seaweed (soak in bath 10 minutes before bathing) and a toning splash for the body. Extra for itchy or sunburnt skin — bicarbonate of soda (3 cups per bath). Put all items in beautiful jars — even oatmeal can look interesting.

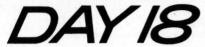
DIET

Breakfast:
½ cup natural yogurt
2 slices melon
1 slice whole-grain toast
coffee or tea

Lunch:
½ cup cottage cheese
1 mixed green salad with ½ teaspoon
    mayonnaise
1 slice whole-grain toast
1 apple
coffee or tea

Dinner:
3 slices roast or boiled chicken, no skin
1 cup finely sliced courgettes (boiled)
1 tomato
½ bunch watercress
coffee or tea

Watercress has often been included in this diet. Make a note of its incredible virtues for now and later. It is one of the finest blood purifiers as it's rich in sulphur, nitrogen and iodine. It is also an excellent source of vitamins A and C, and is good as a general tonic for the liver and kidney. Keep on eating plenty!

Chart Check

Are you making use of the charts? They are daily reminders of what you should be doing and there's no escaping the New You message if they are constantly in view. Make sure they are hung up in obvious places — make sure they are all used.

EXERCISE

In the midst of all your expanding and outgoing activities, there is one controlled movement you should learn. You can do it at any odd moment — standing at the bus-stop, cooking in the kitchen. With it you can achieve a better shape for your buttocks. Stand feet a little apart, slowly draw the buttocks towards each other; when as tight as possible, hold to the count of 6. Relax. You should be using both inside thigh and buttock muscles. Try to make both cheeks pull-in evenly. Initially check in rear mirror in the nude — you'll probably notice that one side moves before the other. Concentrate on it.

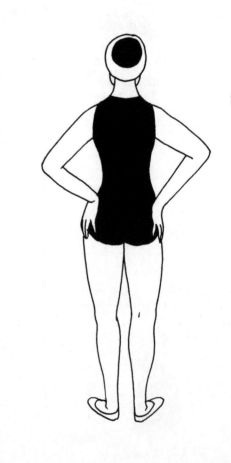

BODY CHECK

Are you easily able to 'switch off' and relax mentally and physically? Most of us are too tense and that ultimately affects all body functions. Here's a technique for mastering relaxation, which can revive you after a few minutes or help you on your way to a good night's sleep. Lie down. Visualize the patterns of your muscles. Send mental messages to them. Here and there contract a muscle, release it slowly — flex a toe, stretch a limb, brace the neck etc, then relax. In this way you will become more conscious of your muscles, where they are, what they do. Now stretch the entire body and hold muscles taut — starting with the feet, through legs and torso and finally to the neck and face. Now in slow motion, let go. Start at the top and work down — relax the head, the jaws, the mouth, the neck, shoulders and so on down to the last toe. End up like a rag doll — through mental willpower.

BEAUTY POINTER

Do you wear perfume every day, all day — or think of it as just a dab here and there on a special occasion? Don't underestimate the value of scent. It's not just a matter of smelling good or bad. The more you learn about fragrance, the more you'll realise how valuable it is. With scent you can create a mood and stir up emotions — and it goes a long way towards creating your personal image, establishing your impact. A woman is often remembered for her perfume as much as her face. So start thinking about it as a necessity. Read all about it on page 91. Flick through the advertisements in magazines so you'll have some knowledge of the various names when you go out to buy. And make a note of this on price: concentrated perfume is very expensive, and in any case can be very overpowering; much less costly are the colognes and toilet waters which are diluted forms of perfume and contain a far higher percentage of alcohol. They are refreshing, they are strong enough to be effective. Start with these — but start on a regular basis.

OPTIONAL

There's little more luxurious than a collection of special toiletries for the bath. The packages are enticing, so are the colours, the scents, the jars. They do important work as well, so they are not that extravagant — prices of the various ranges vary enormously. Look for bubbles, crystals, essences and oils for the bath. Look for body toners, lotions and talcum powders for your body afterwards. But stick to the same fragrance — you'll find many items are coordinated. For greatest effect perfume should be layered: begin with matching scented soap, bath essence, powder and deodorant — then splash on the same perfumed toilet water or cologne.

SKIN CARE

Be independent as regards skin preparations — you never know when it will be necessary — and make your own cleanser and moisturizer. Almond Cleansing Cream: 120g (4 oz) oil of sweet almonds, 30g (1 oz) hydrous lanolin, 30g (1 oz) petroleum jelly (vaseline). Melt fats slowly in a double boiler, remove from heat. Beat until cool. Rose water Moisturizing Lotion: 5 tablespoons glycerine, 3 tablespoons rose water. Pour into a bottle and shake well before each using.

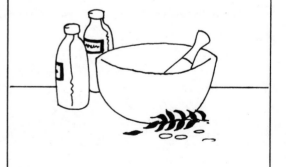

OPTIONAL

You're fast becoming a New You inside and out, so what about treating yourself to some delicious first layers, some fabulous new underwear. Don't think about practical garments, think of a romantic covering, of silk and satin and lace and allure. Go out and find the best. Meanwhile think about what Dorothy Parker reportedly once wrote for a lingerie caption:

There was a little girl, who had a little curl,
Right in the middle of her forehead,
When she was good, she was very, very good,
But when she was bad . . . she was dressed in
*   this ravishing, silk satin, low-necked, lace-*
*   trimmed gown . . .*

BODY CHECK

Is your mind working as well as your body? How's your concentration? Can you concentrate on this book, for instance? Wandering minds are common — and they get worse as one gets older. Learn this mental exercise, use it often and you'll slowly be able to train your brain to register things at will. At first your mind will be fuzzy, but persevere. Walk into a room and be very conscious of the surroundings. Use your mind like a camera. When you leave carefully recall as many scenes from it as possible — places, points, colours, objects, people, actions. Make your mind work — don't give up. It may help to write down everything.

EXERCISE

Whilst walking and exercising think about a sport you'd like to start doing regularly when the 21-day build-up is over. (See page 74 for suggestions.) You now have the stamina and the flexibility. Of all the sports, swimming is the most beneficial all round exercise. It's excellent for breathing and circulation; it strengthens and firms all muscles and helps align the bones of the spine. Indeed, if you have any problems with your back, get in the water right away. Breaststroke is particularly good for back, bosom and legs. Swim at a leisurely pace, don't worry about speed. If you start to swim regularly you'll be amazed at your improvement in only a short time. Measure proficiency by the number of lengths you can complete. Aim to swim for 20-30 minutes 3 times a week. You'll burn up approximately 350 calories an hour.

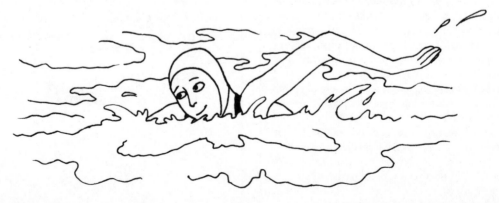

SKIN CARE

If you're going to take up a sport, you need to watch your skin. All elements play havoc with it. In wind and rain you'll need a rich conditioner (even vaseline will do), while in the sun — whether in the snow or in the summer — you need a sunscreen. This protects the skin by copying the function of your own natural screen, melanin. It scatters all light rays that beam on the skin, and also absorbs the harmful wavelengths. Sunscreens come in varying degrees of strength, which are indicated on labels by reference to the sun screen index or 'sun protecting factor' (see page 79 for chart). Check out the various products and look closely at the labelling — there are many that claim to be suntan lotions but don't have any protective elements in them. Sunscreens are useful protectors in the water too, as they form a substantial barrier against the chlorine of the swimming pool and the salt of the sea. After sports, shower the body, clean the face well, not forgetting to moisturize liberally.

BEAUTY POINTER

Perfume buying day: but before you go, check the possibilities, the types of fragrances. Do you want something fresh, flowery, spicy, sexy? Check references on page 91. There are hundreds of different fragrances and the only way to find out which one is for you is to test them, not by buying a whole bottle, but by using the tester samples that are readily available. Don't test more than 2 scents at a time. First smell the scent in the bottle — this is its 'top note'. Next apply a bit to the inside of your wrist — put a different one on each wrist. After half an hour smell again — this is the 'middle note'. Wait another hour, smell once more — this is the 'bottom note'. Consider your reaction to all 'notes', particularly to the 'bottom' one as this lingers on. The reason for doing this is that fragrance varies from when in the bottle to on the skin. Your skin type and chemistry greatly influence the effect — and everyone has a different reaction to a particular fragrance. And don't expect to find the perfect one first time round — carry on testing and testing — and testing.

DIET

Breakfast:
½ grapefruit
1 poached egg
1 slice whole-grain toast, brushed with
   margarine
coffee or tea

Lunch:
125g (4 oz) grilled liver with just a little
   margarine and chopped sage
1 cup sliced green beans
1 tomato
1 slice pineapple
coffee or tea

Dinner:
125g (4 oz) grilled fish
1 large green salad with 1 teaspoon
   mayonnaise
1 slice whole-grain toast
1 slice pineapple
coffee and tea

Sage is a common herb that you've doubtless only thought of in terms of stuffing. Well, it's also great with liver — but more important is its value as a health remedy. Its reputation goes back centuries as a stimulant for the nervous system and brain. It is used by herbalists as a digestive to aid stomach problems that are of nervous origin. You can only gain if you use sage in cooking and drink more sage tea: ½ teaspoon of dried leaves or 2 fresh ones in a cup of boiling water; cover and steep for 5 minutes; sip slowly whilst still hot. A wise man was not called 'sage' for nothing!

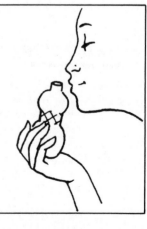

BEAUTY POINTER

Perfume can lift the spirits — make it part of your daily life — make it a personal signature. Spray it on, splash it on. A few warnings: don't overdo it — your nose gets used to a scent after you've worn it for a while, but others are very aware of it. Too much scent can be unpleasant particularly at close quarters. Don't keep scent in direct light. Put bottles in a cool dark place, this helps preserve it. Don't use scent to counteract sweat — the chemical reaction smells dreadful. Don't put scent on clothes. First of all, it might stain and, more important, scent not in direct contact with your skin doesn't take on its individual character. And watch about wearing scent when sunbathing; some scents contain ingredients that have an adverse reaction to direct sunlight and can cause skin irritations and rashes. Other than that, enjoy it.

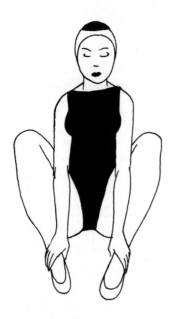
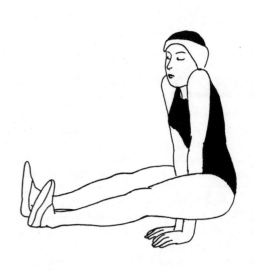

EXERCISE

A test today — to be done after your usual routine. How well can you now control your body? These 2 movements really stretch your ability, stretch endurance. If you can do them — bravo! 1. Scissor Balance — sit, legs slightly apart; lean back to rest on the coccyx; bend knees in order to grip both insteps; straighten, stretch and open legs into a wide scissor movement; really stretch the back of the knees, push hard, hold to the count of 10. Relax. Repeat 5 times. 2. Airborne lift: sit, legs wide apart, arms between legs, palms flat. With weight on hands, lift legs a fraction off floor. Bend legs, stretch and push, bend, stretch and push, continue 10 times without legs or bottom touching the floor.

DIET

Breakfast:
1 slice pineapple
½ cup yogurt
1 slice whole-grain toast, smudge margarine
coffee or tea

Lunch:
½ cup cottage cheese
1 large fruit salad
coffee or tea

Dinner:
125g (4 oz) lean beef steak, grilled
1 baked potato with 2 teaspoons sour cream,
   plus a handful of chopped chives (eat skin)
1 tomato
6 slices cucumber
1 slice pineapple
coffee or tea

A potato is added to the diet today to get across the fact that potatoes in themselves are not fattening such as sugars and fats. They only become fattening when fried. The potato also happens to be one of the most nutritious vegetables, but because the important elements lie just under the skin, the healthy way to eat them is baked or boiled complete with scrubbed skin. They are a useful source of vitamin C, also contain the valuable B vitamins and a rich supply of potassium.

BODY CHECK

Assess your stress level. How? By analysing how tense you are. What aggravates you, when are you most nervous, how jumpy, how quick tempered? Stress levels are individual. We each have a limit as to how much stress we can stand before the brain is alerted and our emotions go into action. Think seriously about what causes you stress and try to work out something positive about it. Anxiety is frequently the main cause, and it is extremely common in women. It is different from fear, which is reaction to definite real danger. Anxiety is a neurotic response, for it anticipates a catastrophe that is usually imagined. Most women who suffer from anxiety are never quite sure exactly what it is they are so anxious about, although when asked will list generalities such as money, the future, security, losing a job, losing a husband, the children, the home, growing old and so on. Are you guilty of worrying about any of these? Do you panic before anything actually happens? The problem is that although you are not worrying about anything specific, such is the power of the imagination that it can direct the brain into action as though real ordeals were imminent — and stress and tension follow. To help control anxiety, try rationing yourself. List the most important things to worry about and concentrate on those. It sounds odd, but it works. Try to live from day to day; don't look back (the 'if only' syndrome) and don't peer into the future. Get a grip of yourself — for today, make a limited worry list and stick to it.

OPTIONAL

Can you afford some marvellous new clothes now that there's a marvellous New You to put into them? A shopping expedition when you are feeling and looking super is so rewarding. But don't run out without a thought. First take a long look at yourself — at your shape, your type, your style, your desired image. Then take a long look at magazines — work out what you like, what's for you, what colour. Now a long look at windows and a long walk through the shops. It's the only way to successful dressing. After all this, decide and spend and revel in it.

SKIN CARE

Have you bought a bottle of rose water yet? Do so. It is a main ingredient for many of the simple home-made recipes, and on its own it's a treasure of a skincare product. It is available inexpensively at most chemists. As is, it's a valid skin freshener; with witch hazel (see page 27) it's a great toner; with glycerine (see page 47) it's a moisturizer. It can scent a bath, be added to handcream, be used as a body splash after the bath. It's been prized for generations; don't overlook its value today.

DAY 21 ● The finishing post — HURRAH!

DIET

Breakfast:
1 bowl of strawberries or raspberries
½ cup natural yogurt
1 slice whole-grain toast with smudge margarine
coffee or tea

Lunch:
2 hard boiled eggs
1 tomato
1 large green salad, ½ teaspoon mayonnaise
(chop eggs and tomato and put on salad)
1 slice whole-grain toast
coffee or tea

Dinner:
3 slices roast lean lamb or turkey without skin
¼ cup boiled brown rice
1 cup green string beans (sliced)
1 tomato
1 bowl of strawberries or raspberries

How well have you been sticking to this diet? If you've been rigid, you'll have lost weight and be feeling fitter. Hopefully you will also have got into the habit of eating fresh foods, balancing your diet and not snacking between meals. Don't revert to old routines. Continue eating healthily, eat more — though not that much more — but eat the same sort of foods. Check the 'Maintenance Diet' on page 62. And drinking? In moderation it is just fine, never did anyone any harm. Wine with meals, a controlled amount of spirits at other times. Enjoy your food, it's one of the great pleasures of life.

EXERCISE

No slacking on the last day please. But then this isn't the final day for exercise is it? You must be feeling so much happier with your new shape, so continue what you have striven so hard to achieve. Sit down right now and make a list of your exercise plan for the next month. How much walking, cycling, skipping? When are you going to do your daily calisthenics? Are you going to take up a sport? Which extra movements did you like most — the Yoga postures? Which are you going to make your daily musts? Today just run through all those Yoga ideas — the breathing, the morning stretch, the shoulder stand, the relaxing poses.

BEAUTY POINTER

Manicure and pedicure day — you should be getting quite adept at it. Do you think you originally chose the right colours? Perhaps a change next week would be a good idea. Get yourself ready for an evening celebration — after 21 days you deserve it. Can you now get the best face in 7 minutes flat? Do you know exactly how your hair should look for maximum effect and flattery? Don't just do a mental check on whether you are pleased or not with your beauty efforts. Make another list — pop it in your personal beauty file. Draw up 2 columns, one headed 'right' and the other 'wrong'. Be honest, deluding yourself is no way to a successful image. You may need to make more adjustments.

SKIN CARE

It's the day of rest again, so give yourself a steam facial (see page 24) or repeat last week's conditioning mask if your skin is particularly dry. No make-up afterwards, of course. After 3 weeks of trying and making several products, going through many procedures, which are you going to make regular, dutiful habits — for you and your skin? Never, never stop the cleanse/tone/moisturizer routine. But how often do you think you need a facial, a special conditioner, a night cream? And can you do the skin-stroking movements without looking?

BODY CHECK

A nice long soaking bath today — in oatmeal, in powdered milk, in your favourite essence, bubbles or herbs. Do bath exercises, foot exercises, hand exercises. Remember them? If not refer back to page 19 and page 35 and page 23. Realistically judge your body in the mirror. How much sleeker does it look than 3 weeks ago? Can you quickly run from top to toe and know at once what treatments can improve any area, any problem? Do you know what it needs every day — how much friction, how much exercise, how much conditioning? When did you last check on superfluous hair? Maybe not since that first day. Do so right now.

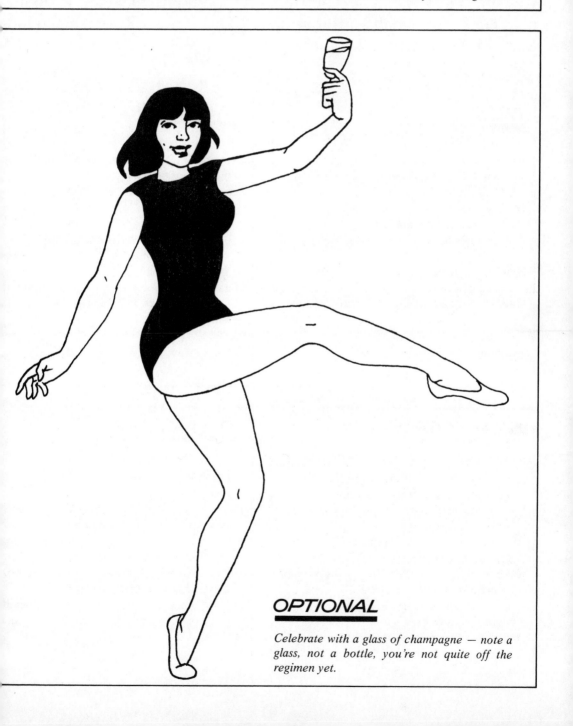

OPTIONAL

Celebrate with a glass of champagne — note a glass, not a bottle, you're not quite off the regimen yet.

CHECK OUT

It's 21 days since you completed the CHECK IN questionnaire. No[w]
how do you feel? How do you look? Has your attitude toward[s]
yourself and your health and beauty potential changed? It couldn[']
help but be drastically different if you stayed the full course. To judg[e]
how you fared, here's another quick test.

DIET

Have you followed the diet exactly?

Are you paying more attention to the value of fresh food?

Have you got into the habit of cutting out sugar and cutting down fats?

Are you going to continue to avoid fried foods?

Have you started using more herbs? For cooking? For teas?

Have you decided it's best to limit alcohol?

EXERCISE

Do you feel you have really benefited from the exercises?

Have you planned an exercise programme for the future?

Are you going to aim for a minimum of ½ hour outdoors activity every day?

Are you now well attuned to the variou[s] Yoga postures?

Have you learned to snatch odd moment[s] during the day to quickly do a specia[l] exercise?

SKIN CARE

Are you now absolutely sure about your particular skin and its special needs?

Do you automatically do the daily cleanse/tone/moisturize routine?

Are you going to continue to exfoliate your skin with salt once a week?

Have you got into the habit of a weekly steam or conditioning facial?

Have you established whether you need a night cream or not?

Have you tried making and using any of the home-made natural preparations?

BODY CHECK

Have you made all your medical appoint[t]ments for checkups?

Have you learned how to relax properly[?] How to revive in 10 minutes?

Have you got a new positive attitude toward[s] taking care of your feet?

Are you trying to protect your hands from the elements, particularly water?

Have you mastered the technique of cleanin[g] teeth efficiently? Are you using denta[l] floss?

BEAUTY POINTER

s your make-up equipment in perfect order?
   The tools? The products?

Have you changed your face at all?

Can you now apply make-up with confidence
   and a sure hand — and quickly?

Are you perfectly happy with your cosmetic
   colours?

s your hair the most successful style ever?
   Colour right?

Are your nails beautifully manicured and
   perfectly polished?

Have you discovered the unique scent for
   you?

Are you wearing scent all the time?

OPTIONAL

Have you been to a health shop yet?

Did you check out local gymns and health
   clubs for their facilities?

Have you visited a beautician for a skin
   inspection and deep cleansing facial?

Are you going to have regular massage
   treatments?

Have you treated yourself to a day of beauty
   in a salon?

Are there some marvellous new clothes
   hanging in your closet?

NEW YOU DATA

Weight: _____

Measurements:

Bust _____

Waist _____

Hips _____

Thighs _____

Knees _____

Calves _____

Upper arms _____

	Good	Much Improved	The Same
General fitness:	Good ___	Much Improved ___	The Same ___
Figure:	Good ___	Much Improved ___	The Same ___
Diet habits:	Good ___	Much Improved ___	The Same ___
Skin condition:	Good ___	Much Improved ___	The Same ___
Make-up:	Good ___	Much Improved ___	The Same ___
Hair condition:	Good ___	Much Improved ___	The Same ___
Hairstyle:	Good ___	Much Improved ___	The Same ___
Hands and nails:	Good ___	Much Improved ___	The Same ___
Emotional state:	Good ___	Much Improved ___	The Same ___

you have answered 'YES' to most of the questions, you are a
formed person . . . you are very definitely a NEW YOU.

ALL THE

EXTRA DETAILS

Diet
ground rules
recipes
energy drinks
maintenance diet

Exercise
First Week Exercise Plan
Second Week Exercise Plan

Sport
clothing check
fitness sports
social sports

Skin
types of skin
basic preparations
common problems
sun and skin
unwanted hair

Manicure

Pedicure

Feet
common problems

Make-Up
glossary of products
equipment basics

Scent

Hair
care and attention
establishing type
style and equipment
change in colour and pattern

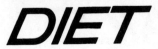

DIET

A successful slimming plan depends on 3 things: the number of calories you consume daily, the type of food you eat and your will to carry it through to the end. In the 21-day regimen, everything has been worked out exactly; you don't have to make any decisions as to the type of food or the quantity. Don't play around with it, because it's balanced to ensure you get a good supply of vitamins and minerals, and it contains a lot of the important high fibre foods.

Ground rules to follow

- never use sugar
- keep salt to a minimum
- no butter; use margarine and oils only when indicated
- all food must be fresh; don't substitute with frozen or canned varieties
- daily milk allowance — 2 tablespoons skimmed milk or 1 tablespoon full milk

Cooking rules

- cooking time for all dishes is short
- vegetables are best steamed, but if boiled do so in little water and for a minimum time
- don't fry anything; meat, poultry and fish can be grilled or roasted in the oven, sometimes boiled or steamed.
- cut away all fat from meat and poultry; don't eat skin.
- all herbs can be used for imaginative flavouring

Drinking rules

- on rising each day, take juice of one lemon in a cup of warm water. This can also be repeated during the day.
- try to drink 575ml (1 pint) of water a day, more is better
- no alcohol at all, no soft drinks
- tea or coffee are allowed anytime and in any amount, but if you add milk keep within the allowance.

The great slimming asset: the lemon

This is your most versatile fruit. Apart from drinking the juice with water, use it to give flavour to meat, poultry and fish; squeeze it over salads and raw foods — even over other fruits. It is also exceedingly valuable as a health food.

Herbal teas for a change

While dieting, the inclination is to drink more as a substitute for food. Excess tea or coffee won't hinder slimming, but neither are very healthy. A good idea is to start exploring various herbal teas. Many taste great, if somewhat unusual, and all provide health benefits. You don't have to go out and buy packaged teas, you can make your own. Simply pour boiling water over the herb and let it steep for a minimum of 5 minutes. Strength is a personal choice, but the average measurement is 15g (½ oz) of the herb to 575ml (1 pint) water. Common herbs can be found at the grocer (or in the garden) others at health food shops. Some suggestions:

basil — aromatic, tasty, it has a calming effect on the nervous system

camomile — one of the most popular herbs, it's calming and has the capacity to induce sleep

mint — refreshing, helps any trouble with indigestion, also good for headaches and generally perks you up

parsley — so common that it is underrated as a health aid, but it is actually rich in iron, calcium, vitamins and trace minerals, and it contains more vitamin C than other common vegetables

rosemary — a strong stimulant, helps both the nervous and digestive systems

sage — also a stimulant, but prime use is as a digestive. For thousands of years, the Chinese have believed in the overall benefits of drinking sage tea daily.

Two special tisanes — one for slimming, one for sleeping

Slimming Tea

Equal parts of: verbena, thyme, mallow, sage, orange blossom. Mix well and use 1 heaped tablespoon to a cup of boiling water; infuse for 10 minutes.

Sleeping Tea

25g (1 oz) dried peppermint leaves, 1 tablespoon fresh rosemary (or ½ tablespoon dried), 1 teaspoon chopped fresh sage (½ teaspoon dried). Mix well together and use 1 good teaspoon to a cup of boiling water; allow to infuse for 5 minutes. Drink just before going to bed.

Basic Recipes for Slimming

When diets refer to whole-grain bread, it means all grains are on the accepted list — wheat, maize, rye and oats. Sometimes they are called whole-wheat or whole-meal loaves. The important thing is that unrefined flours are used. Here's a reliable recipe:

Whole-meal Bread
700g (1½ lb) whole-wheat flour
1 dessertspoon salt
½ cup vegetable oil
½ cup honey
450ml (¾ pint) warm water
15g (½ oz) fresh yeast or 2 teaspoons dried yeast

Mix the flour, salt and oil in a large bowl; in another bowl put the honey, pour over the warm water and stir in the yeast. If dried yeast is used, leave for 15 minutes to activate. Make a hole in the flour and pour in the yeast and honey mixture. Blend until a firm dough is formed. Knead on a floured surface for about 10 minutes. Form a ball with the dough, place in a covered greased bowl and leave in a warm place to rise for an hour — the dough should double in size. Knead for another couple of minutes; shape into a loaf and put in a greased 1kg (2 lb) tin; cover and leave until it has reached the top of the tin. Bake in a hot oven (450°F, 230°C, Gas 8) for 10 minutes, then lower the heat to 400°F (200°C, Gas 6) and bake for a further 20 minutes, or until cooked through.

Every now and then, even when not on a diet, it is a good idea to have 2 or 3 days eating only vegetables and fruits. The following vegetable soup provides a substantial meal:

Vegetable Soup
1 cup chopped onions
3 stalks celery, chopped
1¾ litres (3 pints) water
2 potatoes, chopped small
4 carrots, sliced
sea salt and pepper
1 cup chopped root vegetable
1 cup coarsely chopped leafy vegetable — spinach, broccoli etc

Put a smear of vegetable oil into a large pan, braise the onions and celery just a little. Add the water and then the other vegetables except the leafy one. Season with a little sea salt and lots of fresh ground pepper. Bring to the boil, then simmer for 30 minutes, now add the leafy vegetable, chopped. Cook for a further 3 to 5 minutes.

Eat Right Guide for After 21-Day diet

Hopefully, following the diet has made you think more about the value of certain foods. Now you can eat more, but the same principles of the type of food, and the way you cook it, still apply.

The Important details

• *make time for breakfast* — it really does make a difference if you start the day with a good breakfast. Also eating fruit in the morning wakes you up. Suggestions are — grapefruit, orange, melon, berries. All these provide vitamin C. Soft boiled eggs give you iron and the B vitamins. A piece of cheese can provide protein and calcium. Whole-grain bread and honey give you energy. The best breakfast food is this:

Muesli
2 tablespoons oats
juice of 1 lemon
a little milk
2 tablespoons wheatgerm
4 tablespoons water
2 tablespoons honey

Soak the oats overnight in water. In the morning add lemon juice, honey and wheatgerm , mix well. Add the milk, mix. Then on top pile on any fresh fruit — shredded apple is particularly good. You can also add raisins, nuts and, finally, some natural yogurt.

• *beware of snacks* — chips, biscuits, cakes, buns etc are high in fats, sugars, calories, additives and salts. Try to stop eating them. Instead try fruit, cheese, raisins, nuts.

• *the need for fibre* — it's the rough part of food, in fact it used to be called roughage, that your body can't digest. It's very useful, however, because it provides bulk, which means you often eat less because it fills you up. It also helps food to work its way faster through the digestive system. Good fibre foods are: whole-grain breads, bran, sweetcorn, greens, berries, beans, peas.

● *drinks for energy* — instead of taking tea or coffee to perk you up, try one of these:

Super-Health Drink

2 cups yogurt
¾ cup milk
3 tablespoons freshly chopped spinach
1 tablespoon frozen tomato concentrate
2 teaspoons wheatgerm
1 teaspoon brewer's yeast
2 egg yolks
1 teaspoon ground almonds
juice of 1 lemon
juice of 1 orange
1 tablespoon chopped parsley

Mix all together in a blender; chill before drinking. This is so nutritious you can actually have it instead of a meal.

Apple Juice Plus

1 cup apple juice
1 tablespoon dried milk
1 tablespoon ground almonds
1 teaspoon wheatgerm
1 teaspoon brewer's yeast
1 teaspoon honey
1 banana
Mix together in a blender, chill.

Your basic daily plan

Here is a good maintenance diet indicating foods but not quantities. It's up to you to judge what's enough and what's just too much. You don't need scales or calorie counters. You need good sense and a disciplined eye.

It's simpler to think of food in terms of coordinated groups rather than the more difficult references of protein, carbohydrate and fats. There are 5 important divisions — listed below together with how much is ideal each day.

FOOD TYPE	AMOUNT
1. Vegetables and fruits	5 servings daily
Vegetables: those with intense colour — bright greens and oranges are the most nutritious — broccoli, spinach, kale, sprouts, cabbage, green peppers, dark salad greens, alfalfa sprouts, turnips, carrots, potatoes with skin, tomatoes Fruits: the berry group are excellent food value — strawberries, blackberries, blackcurrants, also apricots, the citrus fruits — orange, lemon, grapefruit, peaches, melon, pineapple.	A serving is about 1 cup of vegetables. For fruits, one of medium size, a cup of berries, a quarter of a melon, 2 slices pineapple.
2. Grains, cereals, beans and seeds	4 servings daily
Grains: whole-grain breads, pasta, oats, brown rice Beans and seeds: all seed beans, fresh or dried, lentils	A serving is about 1 cup of cooked grains, 2 slices bread, ½ cup cooked beans or seeds.
3. Dairy products	3 servings daily
Milk: hot or cold Eggs: raw or cooked Cheese: hard varieties are best, also cottage cheese Yogurt: natural low-fat	A serving is a glass of milk, one egg, 55g (2 oz) cheese, 1 carton yogurt.
4. Meat, poultry, fish and nuts	2 servings daily
Meat: liver, kidney, lean veal, lamb, beef Poultry: chicken and turkey Fish: number one choice in this group, all varieties, also shellfish Nuts: peanuts, pine nuts, almonds	A serving is 125-150g (4-6 oz) of fish, poultry or lean meat. ½ cup nuts
5. Fats and sweets	minimum amount

These are pleasure foods and should be considered as rewards but only if you have included the above basics. Food in this group are high in calories and low in nutrients. Take a little butter for bread, sugar or honey if you need sweetening, vegetable oil for cooking and salads. Cakes and sweets should be rare treats.

EXERCISE

FIRST WEEK EXERCISE PLAN

WARM UP — *Stand with legs apart, legs straight, arms held hig[h] over head, hands stretching upwards. Push up the spine, stretch[ing] the back of the neck. Now bend over by pushing bottom out, relaxing arms but keeping legs straight; curl over as far as you c[an] next swing upward to a midway level, then swing down so that arms go through the legs — and swiftly swing up again to the original position. Start by doing 10 times and during the week work up to 20.*

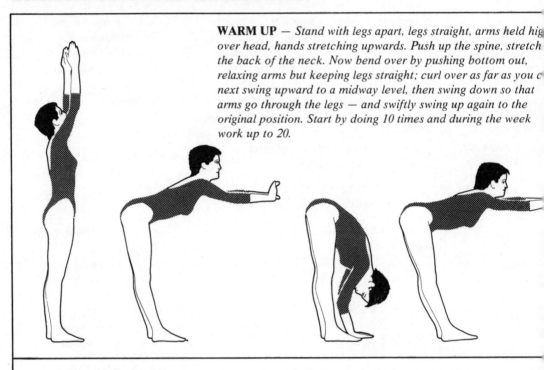

WAIST AND TORSO — *Stand with feet a little apart and clasp hands behind head. Keeping your back straight and elbows well back, bend first to the right, straighten up then bend to the left. Repeat 20 times.*

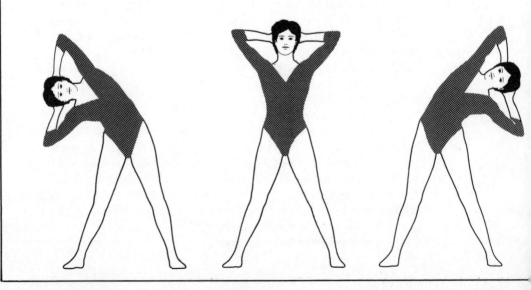

iscipline yourself to 20 minutes a day. It is better to establish a specific time each y — you are more likely to stick to it. These first exercises are easy to do, not o strenuous but very effective if performed regularly. Find the right space; open window. Think of what you are aiming to achieve; think of your muscles — entally visualise which ones you are using and make them work. It is muscle ontrol that can finally change your shape.

HIPS — *Kneel on floor with arms in an arch position over the head, back straight, shoulders down. Really stretch the spine, pulling upwards, then lower hips to touch the floor on the left, then swing to the right, then back and forth 20 times.*

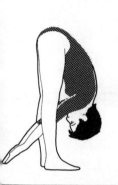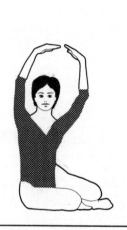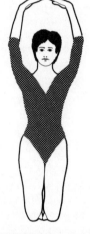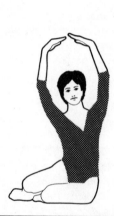

LEGS — *Stand holding onto a firm support at a height comfortable for your arm, feet and legs together, the other arm held out at shoulder level. Swing outside leg back then high to the front keeping torso as rigid as possible — just move the leg, don't twist the rest of the body. Swing back and forth 20 times. Repeat with the other leg.*

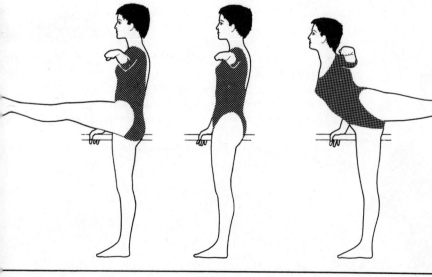

LEGS — *Lie on your left side, using left arm to support your head, place right arm, palm down, in front for balance. Start with legs together, toes pointed, then slowly raise the right leg as high as possible, trying to keep the knees straight — hold to the count of five, then lower very very slowly using the inside thigh muscle for control. Repeat 10 times. Work the other leg on the other side, the same way.*

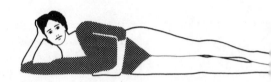

THIGHS — *Lie on back, arms stretched out at sides, palms down. Raise legs until at right angles to the torso, hold together, knees straight, toes pointed. Slowly spread legs to the widest point, hold to the count of 5 then very slowly draw together, making the inside thigh muscles work hard. Repeat as continuously as you can 20 times.*

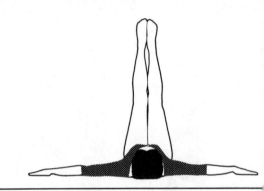

STOMACH — *Lie on your back and tuck feet under a firm, low surface, such as a bed or a couch, and grip it with your toes; knees should be slightly bent. With hands resting on the stomach, raise and lower yourself three times, feeling the pull on tummy muscles. Rest to the count of 10. Repeat 5 times.*

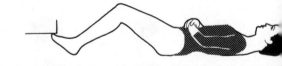

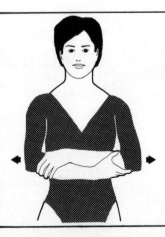

BOSOM — *Stand with feet a little apart and fold your arms, grasping each arm below the elbow with the opposite hand. Push hands towards the elbows — a strong, firm thrust. If you are doing it correctly, you will feel the muscles under the bosom give a definite jerk. Push 20 times.*

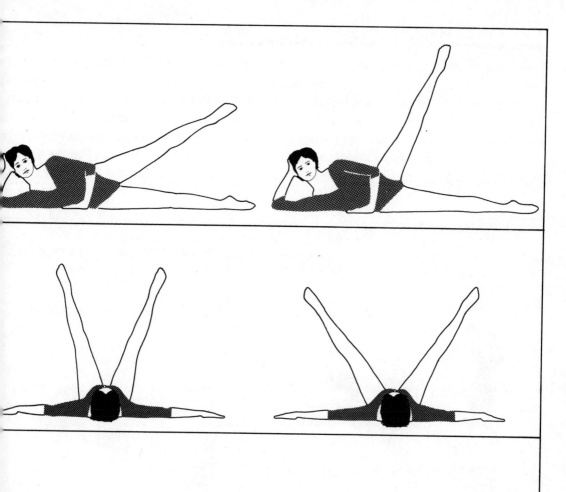

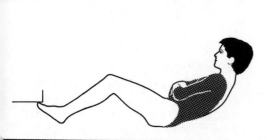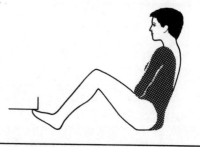

WAIST — *Lie on back with legs bent, knees and feet together; arms should be straight at sides, hands with palms down. At the same time stretch right leg and point toe, and lift* *arm to stretch above the head; really push in both directions and hold to the count of 5. Work alternate sides, six times each.*

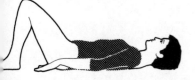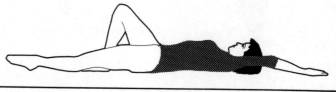

SECOND WEEK EXERCISE PLAN

This programme requires more stamina than last week's. Now your body has g
into the habit of making muscles work, but you're still not at the stage where it ca
be really pushed during a work-out. In addition to the usual warm up sequence, it
a good idea to quickly run through last week's series — then onto the new. If yo
can manage to put in more time than the essential 20 minutes, so much the bette
Some exercises are shown with weights. It is not essential to use them, but th
extra burden does make the muscles work harder and can shape and firm the bod
quicker.

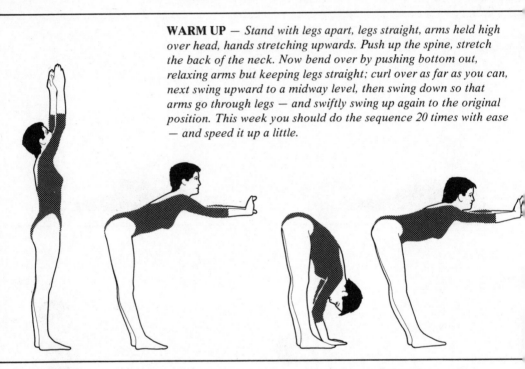

WARM UP — *Stand with legs apart, legs straight, arms held high over head, hands stretching upwards. Push up the spine, stretch the back of the neck. Now bend over by pushing bottom out, relaxing arms but keeping legs straight; curl over as far as you can, next swing upward to a midway level, then swing down so that arms go through legs — and swiftly swing up again to the original position. This week you should do the sequence 20 times with ease — and speed it up a little.*

THIGHS — *Holding onto a support, put your body in a crouch position, heels together, buttocks almost touching heels, roll the pelvis under and keep back straight. Make sure you are balanced on your toes and then bounce up and down lifting buttocks from heels and remaining on your toes. At first do this 10 times and over the week try to work up to 20.*

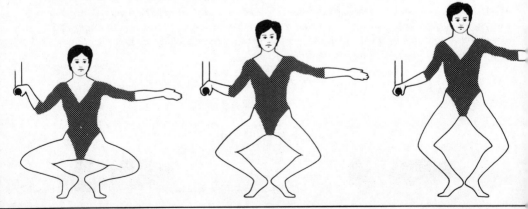

The programme for the final week — and for every day thereafter — is outlined on a special wall chart (loose with the book). Keep it, hang it up, use it each day. You should by now have reached a level of fitness, endurance and stamina that enables you to manage these routines. Initially, however, they are not going to seem that easy. The aim is to gradually push yourself to do them absolutely perfectly, with precise muscle control. If you achieve this, your body will finally reach its best possible shape (remember that means within the limits of body type and bone structure). Continued daily exercise can keep it that way.

WAIST — *With or without weights (books can be used instead) stand with feet together, legs straight, arms at sides, shoulders down, head held high. Slightly flex the knees and pull the right arm up and bend body as far to the left as you can without moving the position of the torso; then lower the right arm and lift the left. Repeat 10 times.*

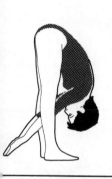
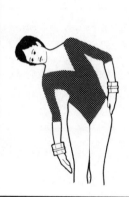
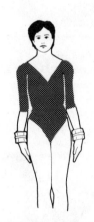
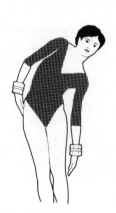

BOSOM — *Stand with legs slightly apart, knees relaxed. Bend over until torso is at right angles to your legs; raise arms to shoulder level and do 20 crawl strokes.*

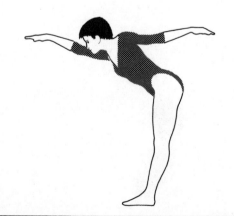
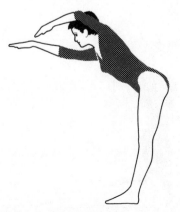

LEGS — *Using weights if possible (the kind that wrap around the ankles), lie flat on the floor on your stomach, arms at sides, legs together, feet pointed. Raise the left leg* *slowly and as high as possible; hold to the count of 10, lower slowly. Do the same with the right leg. Working alternatively, repeat 8 times each leg.*

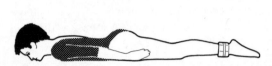 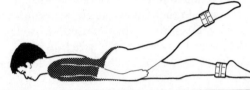

THIGHS — *Lie on back, knees bent and legs together, arms at sides, palms down. Raise your pelvis off the ground and hold to the count of 5, then raise your left leg so that it's* *straight and parallel to the thigh of the other leg; hold to the count of 5. Return to second position; repeat 3 times. Do the same with the other leg.*

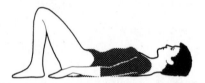 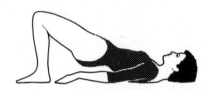

BUTTOCKS — *Start with a kneeling position on all fours (not illustrated) knees a little apart, palms flat on ground. From there lift the left leg, bend arms and raise leg higher putting your body in a slanting line.* Straighten arms and lower leg, now bend arms, lift leg — continue to seesaw in this manner 10 times. Return to kneeling on all fours. Do the same with the other leg.

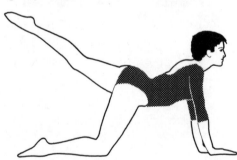 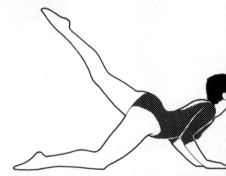

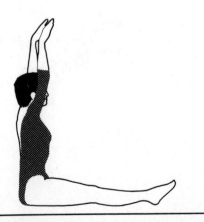 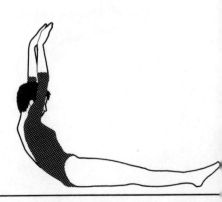

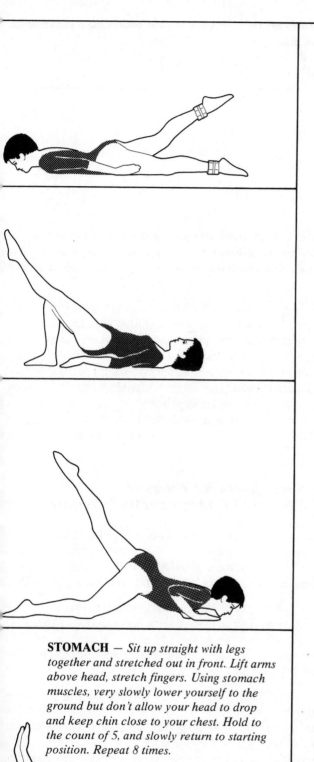

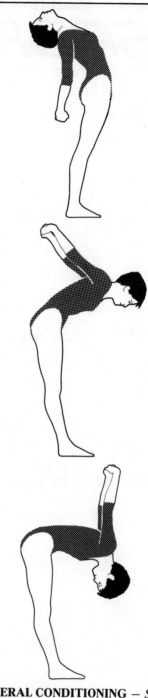

STOMACH — *Sit up straight with legs together and stretched out in front. Lift arms above head, stretch fingers. Using stomach muscles, very slowly lower yourself to the ground but don't allow your head to drop and keep chin close to your chest. Hold to the count of 5, and slowly return to starting position. Repeat 8 times.*

GENERAL CONDITIONING — *Stand with legs a little apart, knees slightly relaxed but not bent at all. Clasp hands behind back and arch the body backwards as far as possible, throwing the head back too; then swing up and over to a forward bend, dropping your head and pushing your arms up as high as possible; hold to the count of 5. Repeat 5 times.*

SPORT

One point to establish from the start: sports keep you fit but unless you are going to devote hours to them every day you are not going to lose weight or get thinner. It's specific exercises that get you trim and keep you that way.

● *check your clothing* — first of all clothes must be comfortable and roomy, nothing tight. Remember you have to move around. And try to wear cotton as it breathes as you sweat and prevents any trapping of moisture. Synthetics can get very clammy and sticky. Wear a bra, again it's best in cotton and with non-stretch straps. All sports require special shoes. Look for layered cushioned soles — avoid synthetics — tops should be canvas, leather or suede, depending on the sport. Go to a specialist sports shop. Try shoes on with the socks you are going to wear. Shoes must fit properly — your feet are very precious.

What are the best sports for fitness?
Walking • jogging • swimming • cycling • tennis

For overall exercise choose one of these. They all are good for building up stamina, for keeping weight under control — and they train the lungs and heart to deliver oxygen-rich blood to the working muscles as fast as possible. Apart from tennis, you can do them on your own.

● *walking* — the simplest way to exercise and maintain health. Do you know that when you walk you use more than half the body's muscles? Aim for an easy continuous motion. Walk briskly — there's no need to walk very fast because it's not the speed that affects fitness, but the endurance of long distance walking on a daily basis.

● *jogging* — fast becoming one of the most popular sports. It is particularly good for heart and lungs and helps to keep you trim. Jogging isn't for everyone and it's not a good idea to take it up in middle age or after if you've not been accustomed to doing any exercise. You should always begin with warm up exercises (do the First Week Exercise series). At first just jog until you are tired — which might not be very far, then walk until you feel up to jogging again. You should never push yourself. Build up stamina and capacity gradually. Jog for 15 minutes 3 times a week to start with.

• *swimming* — the most all round exercise and a pleasure as well. It is excellent for breathing and circulation. It strengthens and firms all muscles. Again build up endurance slowly — start with 1 length, and every third or fourth visit add another length. There's no need to go fast — you're not aiming to get in any team. It is the continuity that matters for fitness.

• *cycling* — great for the legs as it firms up the muscles and can bring new shape. It helps heart and lungs. Use a conventional straight handlebar bike otherwise your posture might suffer. Cycling can easily become part of your everyday life. Speed is unimportant — a methodical continuous rhythm is the aim, and for a specific time (on the average 30 minutes) 3 or 4 times a week.

• *tennis* — a game of doubles may be more social, but a taxing game of singles is better for fitness — and you burn up more calories. Tennis, like all the others, exercises heart and lungs, but it particularly increases flexibility — it helps stomach muscles, trims the legs. If you can't find a partner, many courts and clubs have practice walls — it's almost equal exercise and a good way to improve your shots as well.

Guide for Fitness Schedules

Sport	Weekly Quota	Calories burnt per hour
Walking	30 minutes daily	300-350
Jogging	15-30 minute sessions 3 or 4 times weekly	350-420
Cycling	20-45 minutes 3 or 4 times weekly	350-550
Tennis	1 hour sessions 2 or 3 times weekly	270-400

Eight Popular Sports

It's a pleasure to be out in company — and it's rewarding for your health to be doing some exercise at the same time. Try one of these:

• *Badminton* — a fast and exhilarating game. You need to be agile because you often have to change direction with great speed, and you have to reach up a lot for those high shots. It builds up your endurance level and is particularly good for strengthening the back and shoulders — and improving posture.

• *Dancing* — not really a sport, but it can be a very energetic pastime. All forms are great exercise — what's more it's very relaxing and eases tension.

• *Golf* — something you can play all your life. The emphasis is on skill and although it exercises arms and shoulders and trims the waist to a degree, the real fitness benefit is from the walking involved.

• *Riding* — another sport that has no age limit — you need a good sense of balance plus skill that you can only learn from a teacher. Don't just get on a horse and ride, you could harm yourself. The physical benefits are not that great, but it's good for the inner calf and thigh and can help to improve posture.

• *Skating* — ice-skating is exhilarating (particularly if done outdoors in crisp air). It's good for mobility, circulation, posture and balance. It helps to shape your body and improve leg muscles. Roller-skating keeps muscles working hard because you are constantly on the move. It is also good for strengthening legs and it certainly improves balance.

• *Skiing* — a great sport and one of the best for all round fitness. It is very important to be in shape before you start — ankles, knees and the pelvis structure must be flexible. You also need a good sense of balance. It involves the whole body — you have to twist, turn, bend, pull up, push and control.

• *Squash* — one of the fastest games and it makes heavy demands on your stamina and endurance. It is a game only for those with a high level of fitness. It will certainly keep you trim, make you more supple and faster on your feet.

• *Water-skiing* — almost as good as skiing, but you need to have a strong back and strong arm muscles. It's very good for the legs and for shaping the bottom as you really have to pull in those thigh muscles and hold them taut all the time.

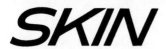

SKIN

Whatever your skin needs in the way of treatment and preparations depends upon its type — and that depends upon texture, colour and condition.

● *Texture: oily, dry or balanced?* Oily skin is caused by overproduction of sebum by the oil glands. It affects darker skins mostly — and most teenagers have oily skins. Skin shines constantly, is often coarse-looking and has enlarged pores. One positive thing — it improves with age, and it stays younger-looking longer. Dry skin is most common in light skins. It is generally of a fine texture, but looks and feels tight. It chaps, flakes and peels easily, and even at an early age may show lines and wrinkles. Balanced skin is extremely rare and only exists when oil, moisture and the skin's acid mantle are all in harmony. It means your skin is quite perfect. More often than not most women have what is known as 'combination skin'. This means the face is usually dry around the eyes and on the cheeks, but gives off too much oil in the T-area of forehead, nose and chin.

● *Colour: light, medium, dark?* The colour of skin depends entirely on the degree of pigmentation — and that depends on heredity. The grades of colour, however, are vast. Light skins go from pale to pink, beige to rosy. Dark skins are graded from olive to caramel, brown to black. The term 'black' however covers a much wider range than 'white'. One skin specialist came up with 35 variations of black skin and only 10 of white.

● *Condition: sensitive or blemished?* Dry skins are usually sensitive — where the skin is fine with a transparent look and likely to develop broken capillaries. Sensitive skins react quickly to climate extremes of heat, cold and wind — and you need to watch out for allergic reactions. Oily skins are usually the ones that develop blemishes — they can be troubled with pimples and spots, often acne.

Taking care of Your Skin

Body skin can usually take care of itself, given daily baths and kept moist with body lotion. Facial skin is more fragile, more exposed to the elements, so its needs are special. It is important not to disturb the skin's normal function any more than you have to. Keeping skin in good condition often means doing less not more. You need a daily routine of cleansing, toning and moisturizing. If your skin is dry you may need a night cream. Once a week skin should be exfoliated — that is the removal of dead surface cells, which otherwise would flake and block up the pores. A weekly steam facial is beneficial — and a conditioning mask does a great deal to help skin. This can be done every 2 weeks. Check the Skincare Chart for all details on care and illustrated procedures.

Basic Beauty Kit

You'll need a cleanser, eye make-up remover, toner and moisturizer — in addition you may need a nightcream, eyecream, throat cream and different masks.

● *Cleansers* — there's nothing like soap, but preferably choose a mild, unperfumed one. The modern cleansing bar is totally non-alkaline and is particularly recommended. Then there are foam cleansers, cream, oil and gel cleansers. It's up to you to find which you prefer by trial and error.

● *Eye make-up removers* — these are often necessary because it can be very difficult to remove eye make-up with ordinary soap and water. There are creams, oils and liquids, also pads saturated with a cleanser. Actually baby oil does a good job — and even better, because it's light, is almond oil.

● *Toners* — these remove the last traces of cleanser, close the pores and generally brighten up the face. There are three grades: a freshner which is the simplest — just an aromatic substance dissolved in water, a mild toner which has some alcohol in it which is adequate for most skins, and an astringent which has the highest degree of alcohol and is good for oily skins.

● *Moisturizers* — the most important of all skincare products. A moisturizer doesn't exactly put moisture into the skin, but keeps the skin's natural moisture sealed in by providing a protective film. It is also an excellent base for foundation, making it easier to blend it in.

● *Conditioning creams* — these contain lubricants which aid a dry skin and help combat lines, wrinkles and a generally aging skin. They are often called nightcreams, because most women use them at night — but they can just as easily be used during the day.

● *Eyecreams* — these are less greasy than conditioning creams, often contain finer oil — the eye area is particularly delicate.

● *Throat creams* — not very different from ordinary conditioners, but sometimes a little richer in oils.

● *Masks* — there are 5 types, each with a different action: cleansing, revitalizing (a quick pick-up), conditioning, stimulating (for circulation) and exfoliating (taking away dead cells).

Common Skin Problems

A trained beautician or skin specialist can successfully treat many problems. If the situation is more serious — such as persistent rashes, allergies or acne, you need to see a dermatologist, the medical doctor who specializes in the diagnosis and treatment of skin problems. He is concerned not only with external correction but with the internal workings of the body.

● *Abscess* — all known as a boil, it is a point of inflammation in the skin with a collection of pus. It starts with red swelling and then a core of pus develops in the centre and finally bursts through the skin's surface. It is usually started by bacteria — sometimes when a spot is squeezed and the surface becomes infected.

● *Acne* — this is caused by over-activity of the sebaceous glands; the excess oil cloggs up and irritates the pores. It is a common teenage problem, though it can occur at any age — often due to stress and sometimes caused by birth control pills. Treatment for acne has advanced considerably in recent years. The most significant development has been the use of antibiotics. They suppress the process rather than cure it; it is a treatment that lasts many months and always under medical supervision. Mild acne does respond to home care — there are preparations available at most chemists. However, it is not advisable to play around too long on your own. There is no one treatment which is good for everyone; you will probably need a combination of products, and only a doctor can work that out properly.

● *Allergies* — what does it mean to be allergic? Certain alien things can make the body produce antibodies as a protective measure. This can result in inflammation and rashes, in breathing difficulties, in sweating, streaming of eyes etc. Reaction varies from person to person. The most common allergy is hay-fever, due to contact with grass or flower pollen. You may find you are allergic to some cosmetics, particularly those for the eyes. Look for non-allergic preparations — there are many on the market. The main thing is to avoid what you are allergic to — the allergen. There are treatments including antihistamines which you get from a doctor. You can also be desensitized — making your body immune — but it can be a lengthy and costly process.

● *Blackheads* — oil plugs in the pores that blacken on exposure to air — the black has nothing to do with dirt, it's the result of oxidization. You can squeeze them yourself, but hygiene is imperative — apply pressure around the blackhead with your fingers, not nails. The tiny black plug should pop out. Dab with alcohol and then witch hazel.

● *Blisters* — usually caused by friction or burns. It's an area of fluid under the skin. Never burst a blister as it's the body's way of protecting the raw skin underneath. Should a blister burst, keep it clean and covered until it completely heals.

● *Dermatitis* — also known as eczema, it's inflammation of the skin. Causes can be physical or emotional. It is usually an hereditary disease and signs appear in childhood. The condition comes and goes, but it should be treated by a doctor.

● *Freckles* — small brown spots and flecks that appear mostly on fair skins and particularly on redheads. A freckle is a small collection of pigment cells. Exposure to sunlight encourages more to appear. There's no way to fade freckles.

● *Itching* — many things can make the skin itch from clothing to bites. Try not to scratch because once the skin surface is broken, bacteria can spread infection. Calamine lotion will bring relief, also bicarbonate of soda (2 teaspoons in a cup of warm water.)

● *Moles* — flat or raised brown patches. They are large collections of pigment cells, often containing hairs. There is nothing you can do to prevent them. Some can be removed surgically. Never pluck hairs from a mole. And if you see any changes — in size or colour, or if it becomes inflamed or itchy, see a doctor right away.

● *Pimples* — spots and red pimples are often found on the face and shoulders. They are skin inflammations and little can be done to prevent them. Don't squeeze unless a blackhead or pus is visible. Wait until pus develops, then gently let it out. Dab with alcohol and witch hazel.

● *Warts* — these are a virus infection. They are actually very infectious, so don't pick at a wart otherwise you may develop a colony. Warts usually last a couple of years. The body will gradually build up antibodies that will kill them off. Warts can be frozen off, chemically removed or electrically treated. Surgical removal is considered the last resort.

● *Whiteheads* — these appear as tiny white beads of wax just under the skin and have no way out unless helped. This means opening the pore and ideally should be done by a trained beautician. They don't leave scars.

Watch your skin in the sun

All skins need some kind of protective cream. Extensive exposure to the sun can cause burning, which damages the skin and could very well set you on the way to skin cancer. And another thing — excess sun makes the skin line and wrinkle, causing premature ageing. This doesn't mean that getting a tan is out. It means building up a tan slowly which is a protection in itself against the sun's harmful UVB waves. What you have to guard against is toasting a skin that has not seen the sun for some time.

The only reliable way of doing this is with a sunscreen. Sunscreens come in varying degrees of strength, which are indicated on the label — by reference to the sunscreen index or 'Sun Protection Factor' (SPF). This is done by numbers from 2 to 12. What it means is that you can stay in the sun for those many hours longer than your natural burning point. Very fair, sensitive skins can burn within 10 minutes; average skins usually reach burning point after half an hour, while tougher skins (those that tan easily) are safe up to 40 minutes. Whatever product you use, it should be applied liberally to all exposed areas, and re-applied every 2 or 3 hours. Most vulnerable parts are face (particularly the nose) shoulders, upper chest, backs of knees. Ideally you should use a total sunblock or the highest SPF for your face. Below is a guide to the length of time you can safely stay in the sun relative to your skin type and the strength of the sunscreen.

Sun Safety Chart

Sun Protection Factor	2	4	6	8	10	12
Skin type Fair	—	—	30-60 mins	40-80 mins	45-90 mins	1½-2½ hrs
Medium	30-40 mins	60-80 mins	1½-2 hrs	2-2½ hrs	2½-3 hrs	5-5½ hrs
Dark	50-60 mins	1½-2 hrs	2½-3 hrs	3½-4 hrs	4-4½ hrs	all day
Black		2 hrs	4 hrs	6 hrs	all day	all day	all day

Unwanted Hair — how to deal with it

Everyone has a certain amount of hair on their body — just about everywhere except for palms and soles of the feet. The question is: is it visible enough to bother you? If so, there are several efficient methods of coping with it.

● *Shaving* — it's fast and easy. It's probably the best for underarms. You can also shave legs — most women do — but it's not advisable to shave arms. Never shave upper lip or the breasts. You can safely shave the bikini line. Hair returns more quickly after shaving than after any other method. It doesn't grow more profusely though, as many women think. It does grow in rough because the hairs have been blunted. The ideal time to shave is after a warm bath or shower when the pores are more open and the hair shafts swollen. Safety razors are best. Make sure the blades are absolutely clean. Use soap and water to work up a lather first. Shave in the opposite direction to growth. And remember, in the case of underarms, do not use a deodorant for 24 hours — if you nicked yourself no matter how slightly, it could cause an infection. Dab with a little talcum powder.

● *Depilation* — removing hair by means of a chemical formula. Depilatories come as creams, gels, sprays and foams. They soften and dissolve the hair shaft but have no effect on the roots. They take about 10 to 15 minutes to work. You must make a patch test first, because some products can irritate sensitive skins. They do not prevent hair growth, so the process has to be repeated about once a month. You can use them almost anywhere, but if you are putting them on your face, check the labels to see if you can. If you are using them on the bikini line, watch that the depilatory doesn't get too close to the vaginal area — wear briefs. Also don't use them on your eyebrows, the danger of getting into the eye is too risky. And don't use them on your breasts.

● *Waxing* — hot or cold wax is put on the skin and then pulled or ripped off. It can hurt a lot, and many women can't stand it. But waxing does get at the hair lower down in the follicle than other methods. It leaves the skin very smooth and it does last longer. You can buy wax strips and do it yourself, but it is less painful when done by a beautician.

● *Plucking* — using tweezers to pull out the odd stray hair. It's perfect for eyebrows, for solitary hairs on the face. Leisurely ladies have been known to pluck their legs — but you need an awful lot of time for that! Never pluck hairs from your breast, and never from a mole. Hairs are easier to pluck if you first steam them with a hot washcloth. This helps open the pores — then with tweezers firmly grasp the hair and with a jerk pull it out. It works best when you pull in the direction in which it is growing.

● *Bleaching* — fair hair shows up less than dark, so if you haven't got much hair, this might be the answer. You can bleach anywhere except under the arms. It's a good disguise and lasts from 3 to 6 weeks. There are several very good commercial products on the market. Two warnings: read the instructions extremely carefully and do a patch test first, just in case you happen to be allergic to it. A small area on arm or leg is a good spot for a trial. Wait 24 hours to see if there's any reaction — meaning no inflammation or itchiness. Bleaching is particularly good for facial hair. It can be tedious on the body if you have a large area to cover.

● *Electrolysis* — this is the only permanent hair removal method because the hair root bulb is destroyed. It is extremely valuable for women who have excess hair on their face — removal from other areas is not really valid or practical. Electrolysis has to be done by a qualified technician as it is a very skilled job. The hairs are treated one by one, and in one session there's a limit as to how many hairs can be dealt with. Usually it involves treatment that goes on for weeks and weeks if you have considerable hair to take care of. It is expensive, but it is one of those beauty treatments that is worth it.

MANICURE

1. Remove polish with a cotton ball moistened with oily remover. The professional way to do it is to first press the cotton against the nail to dissolve the polish, then wipe it off slowly with a pressing motion. You will need more than one cotton ball. Also don't use neat acetone — it is very destructive to nails. Use a good oily remover.

2. File the nails using an emery board — absolutely NOT a metal file. Work with long strokes from side to centre. Don't saw away. It is important not to file too low at the corners as this will weaken the nail and encourage breakage. The best shape is an oval — though if your nails are short it's advisable to leave the sides straight as this will give some strength.

3. Massage a little cuticle cream into the base of each nail. This is best done with the index finger. The cream helps soften and loosen the dry skin.

4. Soak nails in warm soapy water for a couple of minutes — use a bath product not detergent. Scrub away dirt with a brush.

5. Wrap cotton wool around an orange stick, and dip into cuticle oil (sometimes it comes with its own applicator) and smear the cuticles.

6. Take another orange stick, wrap cotton wool around it and after dipping into the soapy water, use it to gently lift the cuticle away from the base of the nail. Smooth with finger into a supple curve.

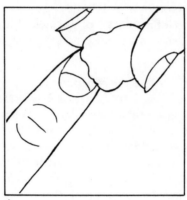
1

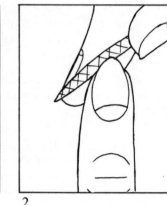
2

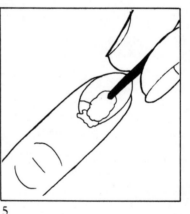
5

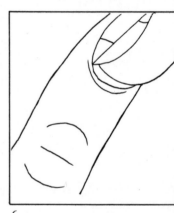
6

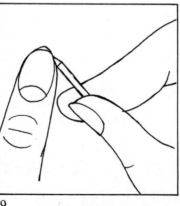
9

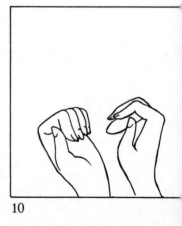
10

Giving a manicure is an acquired skill. If you're new at it, don't expect to get it right the first time. You'll be all thumbs, so to speak. It is important to know the right way to do it. The effort is rewarded by a visual pleasing end. A manicure isn't just a cosmetic treatment for nails. The processes you go through also benefit the health of the hand and nails — it conditions, it stimulates, it protects. Here is the step by step guide — it should take a maximum of 30 minutes, but don't rush it.

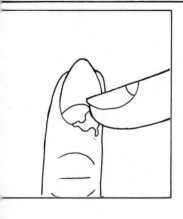

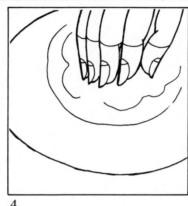

4

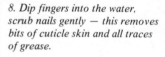

7. Apply hand lotion, don't skimp on it, and massage into hands and fingers giving each finger a good pull from the joint.

8. Dip fingers into the water, scrub nails gently — this removes bits of cuticle skin and all traces of grease.

9. An extra if you want — take a white nail pencil, run the point under each tip. This is advisable if you are not going to wear polish.

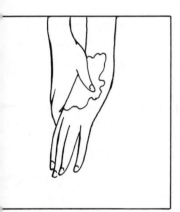

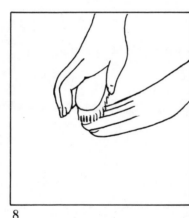

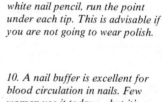

8

10. A nail buffer is excellent for blood circulation in nails. Few women use it today — but it's a definite plus. Buff in one direction only. Also if you don't use polish it's a good idea to use a buffing paste, which helps to condition the nail and also ends up by giving them a marvellous shine.

11. Apply varnish — first a base coat, then 2 layers of colour and if you like a final sealing coat but that is not absolutely necessary. A base coat is the protection layer which prevents polish from discolouring the nail. Apply varnish with 3 straight strokes from the base to the tip — one down the middle, then one either side. Polish the entire nail, it looks better.

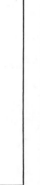

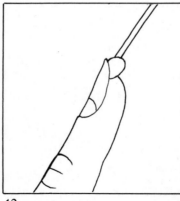

12

12. Check up on smudges — down the sides, over the tip. Wrap an orange stick with cotton wool, dip into remover and run it around the nail and under the tip.

PEDICURE

1. Remove old polish by soaking cotton wool in an oily remover, pressing against the nail, holding for a few seconds and then wiping off.

2. Trim nails — if your big toe-nail is tough you may have to use clippers to cut a straight line across. It is better not to use scissors, even those called 'manicure scissors'. It is important to keep toenails straight — not oval, and certainly not pointed — as this prevents nails from cutting into the flesh. It is also a precaution against the possibility of an ingrowing toe nail.

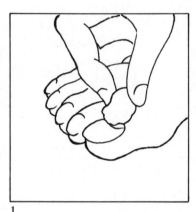

1

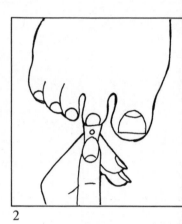

2

3. File nails so they are smooth — file straight across, do not go down the sides.

4. Soak feet in warm soapy water for 5 minutes, more if you like (watch TV or read); now using a bristle brush scrub feet all over, particularly the heel and under-side of the foot.

5. There will probably be several hard and rough spots. These have to be rubbed with a pumice stone or friction pad. If you do this regularly, the lumps will eventually whittle down. When feet are dry they invariably become cracked, particularly around the heel. Dirt gets lodged in the cracks and the only way to remove it is with a pumice stone — and you need to rub a lot. It is not wise to take a razor to your foot to scrape away skin. It is done by some beauticians, but they have the skill to do it efficiently. There are some commercial products for feet that help to get rid of rough skin — try one.

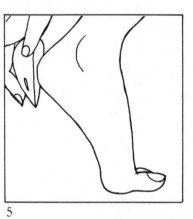

5

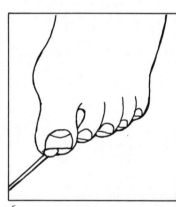

6

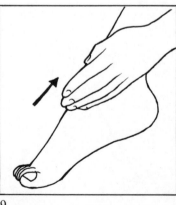

9

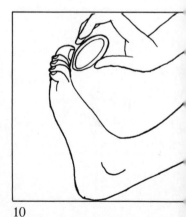

10

It is much more difficult to give yourself a pedicure than a manicure. The basic fact of getting at your feet can be a problem. Fortunately you don't need to do it so often — once every 2 or 3 weeks is usually enough. Feet respond very quickly to attention, which they usually rarely get — and they can look pretty. So learn how to put your best foot forward.

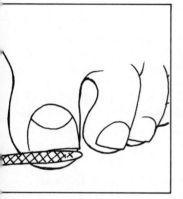

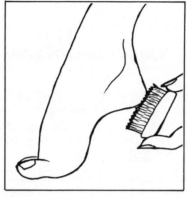

6. Take an orange stick wrap with cotton wool and dip it in the water — then clean thoroughly under the nails, not forgetting to go down the sides.

7. Apply cuticle cream or oil all around the cuticle area; massage gently with a fresh cotton-wrapped orange stick.

8. Rinse foot in water and towel dry — make sure area between toes is properly dry.

4

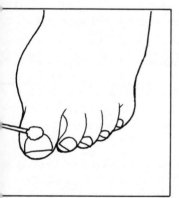

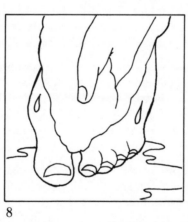

9. Massage in hand or body lotion. Massage all the foot, each toe in turn and then the lower leg with firm upward strokes.

10. Buff nails to help circulation, but in one direction only. Use a buffing paste for a little colour and lots of shine if you are not going to use polish — though coloured toe nails look best as they often have discolourations.

11. Separate toes with a strip of cotton wool or a folded tissue, weaving over and under the toes. This it to make it easier to apply polish and to prevent smudging as toes often press against or fold over each other.

8

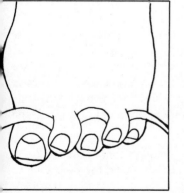

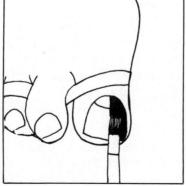

12. Apply first a base coat, then 2 coloured layers of polish. Cover the entire nail — they're small. Clear up any smudge marks using a cotton-wrapped orange stick dipped in remover. Leave for at least 10 minutes to dry before removing the dividing cotton. Leave for another 10 minutes before putting on shoes and stockings.

12

FEET

The most common problems

Most foot problems are due to neglect. Skin builds up due to friction and finally forms bumps and outgrowths which press on nerves or bones and can cause great pain. Professional care is important as most foot problems cannot be taken care of at home.

- *Athlete's foot* — a fungus infection which is usually caught in swimming pools or gyms where people go barefoot. It appears in the form of flaky, itchy skin between the toes — you'll see it easily enough when drying feet. This is one condition you can treat yourself — with medicated liquids and powders from any chemist. However, if the infection persists longer than 2 weeks, go to a chiropodist.

- *Bunions* — a painful lump that usually appears at the side of the big toe. It is caused by badly fitting shoes — too tight or too pointed. It can be helped by foot exercises, but a specialist will give advice on other treatment. The point is that a bunion should be prevented in the first place. Don't ignore it, because if the foot becomes too angled, the only corrective course is surgery.

- *Callouses* — areas of hard, flattened skin, again caused by ill-fitting shoes. They can appear anywhere on the foot, even on the soles. They are less painful than corns, but they can burn to a point of agony. The hard skin can be rubbed down daily with a pumice stone, and gradually you'll wear them away completely. If you are not successful, get professional help.

- *Corns* — these are a build-up of hard, dead skin that appears on the joints. They are almost always caused by tight shoes. The distressing thing about a corn is that it has a point facing inwards and when this presses on a nerve it can be incredibly painful. Wearing a corn plaster can ease the pressure and consequently diminish the pain, but the only way to get rid of a corn is to have it removed by a chiropodist. Don't attempt to cut them down yourself.

- *Ingrowing toenail* — this is when a nail — usually that of the big toe — grows in a curve and digs into the flesh at the side of the nail. Like so many toe problems, this too is terribly painful. It usually happens because the toe has been squashed into tight shoes. You can't do anything about it yourself. Off to a specialist. Sometimes the nail has to be removed.

● *Nail infections* — it's the big toe nail that is more likely to pick up an infection. It is usually caused by a fungus that discolours the nail and thickens it. There are medicated liquid treatments to paint on and under the nail at the tip, also at the cuticle. Quite often the nail has to grow out before it is completely healthy again. It's also common to lose the nail, as the infection lifts it from its base and it becomes quite wobbly. No need to worry though as a new one will quickly grow in its place.

● *Verrucas* — an infectious inward-growing wart picked up by bare feet. Because they grow inward they can be extremely sore. Without professional treatment they will quickly spread. A chiropodist will treat them with an acid product, possibly electronically and in the case of deeply rooted verrucas, surgery is used.

MAKE-UP

How to make it a success

Rule No. 1: get your products right

The essentials you need are: base, blusher, eye make-up colours, eyebrow pencil, mascara, powder, lipstick. You may also need a concealer, highlighter and lipgloss. Here are details on the types of preparations available:

● *Base* — also called a foundation, it's the starting point for everything — it smooths the surface of the skin, gives uniform colour and offers a background for cheek, eye and lip colours.

liquids — give a light coverage. They can be creamy for normal or dry skins or oil-free for greasy skins. They are inclined to be runny and don't give good coverage.

creams — the most popular base and suitable for nearly all skins. They can be applied with fingertips or a sponge.

gels — found mostly in tubes because they squirt out like petroleum jelly. They are natural-looking and good for summer use. They give a workable coverage to the skin and give a coloured sheen to match your tan.

solid cream sticks — the consistency is very thick. They are good for covering up blemishes, but if used all over the face, they give a much too heavily made-up impression.

● *Blusher* — also known as a shader or contourer, though all these are merely modern terms for rouge. To achieve interesting dimensions in a face, a blusher is a valuable cosmetic.

powders — the most popular because with swift strokes of a brush, the face is reshaped in an instant. Powders are compressed and usually come with a wide brush applicator.
creams — applied after the base, blended with fingers
gels — give a glossy look, particularly good on tanned skins.

● *Concealer* — also called a cover-up, because that's precisely what it does — camouflages blemishes, circles under eyes, any skin discolourations. It comes as a very solid cream, also as a stick.

• *Eye Shadow* — vital for today's make-up as it gives colour, shape and dimension to the eye. There are many different types.

powders — pressed into a solid block with a moisturizer added for easier application and cling. Best applied with a brush or sponge applicator. They have good staying power. Powders are popular because you can control the colour and blend it without difficulty. They also give a very natural look.

creams — they are oil-based and blend easily into the skin. Applied with fingertips, they need to be set with a transparent powder otherwise they'll crease.

sticks — more solid than creams, rather like a lipstick, colour is applied directly to the eye area.

pencils and crayons — waxy and wide, they are easy to use and very effective. Colour is drawn on with artistic strokes, but it is important to blend colour in with fingertips. Crayons and powders can be effectively used together.

liquids — emulsions that come in bottles with a brush. Colour is painted on, but it often gives a harsh effect — it's difficult to blend with a liquid.

watercolours — cakes that are applied with a wet brush — as with the liquids, there is trouble with blending — the colour is apt to be rubbed away.

• *Eyebrow Colouring* — pencils are the most popular. The waxy narrow leads need to be sharp to be effective. There are also compressed powders, applied with a slant-edge brush.

• *Eyeliners* — crayons or pencils are the best, though you can also use a watercolour cake and paint with a wet brush.

• *Mascara* — essential to give colour and extra thickness to lashes — without it eyes are lost.

wands — the most popular because they are easy to apply. They contain creams that are rolled on to the lashes with a spiral brush or a screw-like rod. Some contain extra fibres to build-up lash length and thickness.

cakes — block of colour that is rubbed with a wet brush, then brushed on to the lashes. It has to be built up coat by coat.

creams — oil-based and applied with a dry brush, but it's tricky to control and smudges easily.

• *Lip Colour* — all products are formulated to give a moist look. They are a blend of oils, waxes and glycerides, plus colour, perfume and flavour.

lipsticks — conventional form and the most widely used — more effective when applied with a brush.

creams — come in pots, must be applied with a brush.

pencils — soft, wax based — perfect for outlining the lips, not so good for filling-in.

gloss — gives shine but not much colour. Clear gloss can go over ordinary lipsticks — apply with brush or fingertips.

• *Powder* — loose powder is necessary to set make-up and the only one to use is a transparent one. For touch-ups pressed powder comes in compacts.

• *Highlighter* — powder or creams that are pearlized, irridescent with silver or gold flecks — they bring life to the face for the evening. They are applied with a brush or fingertips.

IMPORTANT NOTES

• *Take care of your cosmetics* — keep the lids on and try not to expose products to heat, light, air or moisture. Cosmetics will have a long life if you're careful.

• *Don't share your make-up* — it is possible for infections to be transmitted, particularly through eye products.

• *Watch for allergic reactions* — these are extremely rare, but if your skin is particularly sensitive, it can happen. Change the preparation immediately — look for hypo-allergenic make-up.

Rule No. 2: check on equipment

The accessories you need in order to apply make-up are as important as the preparations themselves. Clean fingers are the best applicators of all, but you also need to assemble the following: handmirror with a magnifier on one side, cottonwool balls, cotton tips, tissues, sponges, sponge applicators for eye make-up, a set of brushes (for eyes, lips, blusher and powder), tweezers, a pencil sharpener and possibly eyelash curlers. And it's easier if you keep them all tidy in a basket or box. Sponges, brushes and applicators must be kept scrupulously clean all the time.

Rule No. 3: acquire technical skill

All the steps to a successful make-up are clearly given on the New You Skincare Chart. Check it out.

SCENT

What do you know about it?

Originally aromatics were single, natural elements, mostly from flowers, leaves and stalks. Today they are complex compounds. It takes many years to create a new perfume and the raw materials come from 3 sources — botanical, animal and chemical. The chemical ingredients are called aldehydes and have been developed over the last 40 years. There are about 3,000 'smells' available to perfumiers.

Finding your way through the labrynth of perfumes can be very confusing, particularly if you are a beginner and are still at the lavender water stage. There is a bewildering variety of scents to choose from. However, perfumes can be grouped into general categories according to their composition and the impression they give:

single floral — the focus is on one 'smell' — a recognizable flower, such as jasmine or violet. They can be sweet or fresh.

floral bouquets — like a bunch of flowers, but the perfumier is also able to mix seasons. Many are a combination of jasmine, tuberose and gardenia. On the whole they are rather sweet.

green — these are the grasses, leaves, ferns and barks. They smell fresh and very woodsy.

citrus — lemon, orange and bergamot feature strongly in this group. They are fresh, cooling and give a tangy impression.

oriental — made from eastern plants and flowers, usually rich in musk and ambergris (animal extracts). They are rich, sweet, often spicy and can be very overpowering.

modern — made from synthetic materials, they represent the feeling of today — they are bright and breezy, fresh, young.

When searching for the right perfume, the only way is to go out and test — and test. The names are mostly rather elusive and give no indication as to what the smell might be, nor what the components are. If you're new at it, try the moderns first, then the single florals.

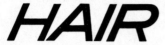

HAIR

Basic Care

Hair should be washed as often as necessary. If hair is oily this could mean every day. Normal or dry hair requires a minimum of 1 wash a week. There are 4 steps to follow — shampooing, rinsing, conditioning and drying. Simple enough, but are you doing them right? Check all the points below:

• shampooing: a pre-rinse is essential, really soak your hair well otherwise you'll never get a good lather from the shampoo. Watch you don't get hair knotted up. Use only a little shampoo. Most people use too much — a tablespoon altogether is usually quite enough. Don't put directly on hair, instead pour a little on to the palm of your hand, rub hands together and then smooth all over your hair. Be gentle — rough handling of hair during washing can cause damage and aggravate any problems. As the shampoo starts to lather, massage the scalp with the tips of your fingers — do so for 2 or 3 minutes. If hair is washed frequently, it will only require 1 shampooing. If it's dirty, it will need another but the first one must be rinsed away before starting again. An important point: if shampoo doesn't lather the first time, don't add more — rinse off and apply another.

• rinsing: hair that is not properly rinsed might just as well not have been washed. The slightest remains of soap will leave hair dull and sticky, attracting dirt immediately — and causes the scalp to itch. Rinse hair for a much longer time than you think is necessary. Rinse, rinse and rinse again with clean running water. Try to make the last rinse of cool water, in fact as cold as you can bear it. If hair is properly rinsed it should squeak when pulled between fingers. You can add a final rinse which is good for all types of hair as it provides an acid mantle, but is particularly beneficial for oily hair:

for dark hair
1 tablespoon of wine or cider vinegar in 1¼ litres (2 pints) of water

for light hair
1 tablespoon of lemon juice in 1¼ litres (2 pints) of water

• conditioning: this is a protective measure and is essential for dry hair. Even if hair is in good condition, a conditioner makes hair softer and more manageable; it helps remove tangles and snarls, gives lustre and controls flyaway hair. If your hair is normal or dry, apply conditioner to the whole head; if it's oily only apply to the ends and only if these are dry or damaged. Apply conditioner to the palms of hands, rub together then gently apply it to the hair. Don't massage it in, but drag fingers through hair working from back to front in the direction of hair growth. If you are conditioning only the ends, soak a cotton ball with conditioner and rub over the tips. Leave on for a minute, gently comb hair starting at the ends, free knots gently. Rinse 2 or 3 times with clean water.

• drying: hair is best dried naturally, first patted with a towel, then combed (never brush wet hair) and adjusted into place. However many styles demand more effort and for greater control it is better to set hair on rollers or blow it with a hand-dryer.

rollers — the bigger the roller, the looser the set. Avoid rollers with brushes inside as these can split hair. Setting lotion can make hair easier to handle. Don't put too much hair on the roller and work in sections of 4-5 cm (1½-2 inches). Hair should be wrapped smoothly, but not tightly, round the roller, first stretching it straight in the opposite direction from which it is to be rolled. Use metal clips to hold in place. Hair can be dried naturally or with a dryer (before taking rollers out allow hair to cool down to room temperature). Take out lower rollers first. When brushing out, brush straight back from root to the tip of strands.

blow-drying — divide hair into 4 sections, secure with clips. Begin drying the back first and dry the roots, then the centre of the strands, then the ends. Next do the sides, finally the crown section. You'll need a circular brush. Don't pull hair too taut, it will cause damage. And watch that the dryer is not too hot, nor so near the scalp that it scorches your hair.

The Right Tools

• brushes — natural bristles are best, but if you choose a nylon one, be sure the ends are rounded. Wide spacing between bristles is important as this makes it easier to get through the hair without causing damage. Rubber cushion brushes are good as they prevent bristles from tugging hair. Flat brushes are for getting out tangles and giving shine. Circular brushes are for styling.

• combs — the perfect comb is one that is saw-cut, which means that each individual tooth is cut into the comb, leaving no rough or sharp edges. Teeth should have rounded tips (not squared off or pointed) that are wide-spaced so that the comb can get through the hair without pulling it. The best ones are made of vulcanite. You can get saw-cut combs made of plastic, but check the tips to be sure as the majority of plastic combs are moulded and have very sharp pointed teeth that are bad for the scalp. Never use a metal comb.

• rollers — the best are: mesh for fine hair, sponge ones for delicate hair and perforated plastic ones for strong and curly hair.

• hairpins — straight big pins for securing rollers or for putting up hair; steel clips for holding rollers and for setting waves and curls; grips for securing hair; pins with concertina section hold complicated styles firmly in place and don't show.

The limits of change

Do you know what type of hair you have? The first step to splendid hair is to be sure of its type and be aware of its limits. Hair has a will of its own and it's a dead end trying to force it to do something unrealistic. Check on 4 points:

• texture — fine or coarse?
• body — thick or thin?
• pattern — straight, wavy or curly?
• colour — good or bad?

Once you've established what your hair is, you are more aware of what you can and cannot do with it — what you should do as well. If your hair is thin, no way are you going to get a voluminous mane out of it. If it's fine you are always going to have trouble keeping its shape. If it's curly, it will be an endless torment if you insist on a straight sleek cut.

Only certain things work. Firstly, there's little to be done about texture and body. Conditioners can help, but that is temporary from wash to wash. When it comes to pattern, the more you go along with the natural tendencies of your hair, the easier it is to take care of — and ultimately the more successful it will be. Whatever you do with curly or wavy hair — short of chemically straightening it — the natural pattern will always return, and only too quickly. Straight hair can be coaxed into waves and curls, can be made to turn up, fold under, but it too will revert to its natural line. Only a permanent wave will ensure a long-lasting effect. Colour is something else — you can definitely do something about it.

Colour: the big difference

Today any hair can be any colour — thanks to modern technology there are easy to use products that offer the promise of instant change. If hair looks wrong, it often has more to do with colour than style. Dull, drab, mousy hair, greying hair, faded hair can negate even the most brilliant cut. Could a new colour make all the difference to you?

There are 3 kinds of haircolouring — temporary, semi-permanent and permanent. It is possible to do all 3 yourself, though naturally a colouring specialist would have the best eye and the professional know-how.

Temporary rinses — these are applied after shampooing hair, often incorporated in the shampoo itself. They only last until the next shampoo. They coat the outside of the hair shaft and because they don't have any bleaching agent, they cannot lighten hair. You can only make subtle changes, adding highlights within your own colour range. Results on colour vary, depending what colour your hair is, but usually packages have clear charts and guides for you to follow.

Semi-permanent tints — these also do not have any bleaching agent, but are stronger than temporary rinses as they contain a chemical that diffuses the hair shaft with a degree of colour. Again, they add highlights within the same colour group. With each shampoo a little colour is washed away. It takes 4 or 5 washings to disappear completely.

Permanent colourings — these contain bleaching and colouring agents. Virtually any colour change is possible. At a salon, the colourist will know exactly what colour and what strength to use to get from your colour to the one you want. If you are doing it yourself, it is a little more tricky. Looking at the colours on the package is only a rough guide, as these indicate how the tint would take on colourless hair. Some products attempt to do more complicated guides, but because everybody's hair is fractionally individual you can never be sure of the results until you've tried it.

Darkening hair is easier than lightening it — it's simpler to gauge the final colour. To lighten hair by more than a few degrees requires pre-bleaching.

If you are doing it at home, you must make 2 tests before colouring the whole head. First a patch test for allergic reactions: make up a small amount of the colouring, wash the skin just behind the ear, swab on some of the mixture and leave on for 24 hours. If there is no sign of inflammation, carry on.

At the same time, do a strand test to check on the colour — cut off a few strands near the scalp and use the rest of the trial mixture. Follow the instructions on the packet — this is most important, as many products have special procedures and timing. Read the labels, follow the guide.

A natural colouring agent: henna

Henna gives a red tint — and is also a good conditioner for hair. But a word of warning: it should be used with caution as you can end up with very strange shades of red. The colour is unpredictable. So never do the whole head without testing first. Read instructions carefully as to quantity and procedure. Hair must be shampooed before using henna. It's advisable to wear gloves, otherwise you'll have red hands too.

What about bleaching?

A bleach strips hair of colour. The most popular one is hydrogen peroxide which comes in different strengths from 10 volume up to 100 volume and the stronger the solution, the faster the action. Bleaching is best done professionally, because if you leave the bleach on too long hair can be very badly damaged. If you do it at home, however, be careful never to use peroxide stronger than 20 volume. The longer the peroxide stays on the hair, the lighter it gets. After bleaching, the hair can be rather yellow and you'll need a colour-rinse to tone it down.

Changing the pattern

Straight hair can be given a permanent, which doesn't necessarily mean lots of waves and curls — that's controlled by the length of time it stays on the hair — but it's often used to help give more body to hair. You can do it at home, the procedure is simple, but you must faithfully follow directions on the packet. Each product has its own directions. Home permanents come in 3 strengths — for fine, medium and coarse hair. Check the labels and match your type.

Straightening hair is perming in reverse, but it should never be attempted at home. It's not that advisable in a salon either as it is potentially damaging.